NOW THAT I HAVE CANCER, I AM
WHOLE

NOW THAT I HAVE CANCER, I AM
WHOLE

REFLECTIONS ON

LIFE AND HEALING

for CANCER PATIENTS

AND THOSE WHO

LOVE THEM

JOHN ROBERT McFARLAND

**Andrews McMeel
Publishing, LLC**
Kansas City

Part I originally published in 1993 under the same title.

07 08 09 10 11 RR2 10 9 8 7 6 5 4 3 2 1

Library of Congress Cataloging-in-Publication Data

McFarland, John Robert
    Now that I have cancer, I am whole : reflections on life and healing for cancer patients and those who love them / John Robert McFarland
      p. cm.
    Includes bibliographical references (p. 297).
    ISBN-13: 978-0-7407-6372-4
    ISBN-10: 0-7407-6372-5
     1. McFarland, John Robert. 2. Cancer—Patients—Religious life. 3. Cancer—Patients—Biography. 4. Cancer—Religious aspects—Christianity. I. Title.

BV4910.33.M34 2007
242'.4—dc22

                         2006052608

www.andrewsmcmeel.com

THIS IS FOR MY WIFE, HELEN KARR McFARLAND,

AND FOR OUR DAUGHTERS,

MARY BETH AND KATHLEEN ANNE.

WITHOUT YOU, I WOULD NOT BE ALIVE.

WITHOUT YOU, I WOULD NEVER HAVE BEEN ALIVE.

AND FOR OUR GRANDDAUGHTER,

BRIGID MARY,

MY MENTOR IN ALL THINGS BRIGHT AND BEAUTIFUL,

and FOR OUR GRANDSON,

JOSEPH PATRICK,

MY HERO.

CONTENTS

PART I:
WHEN YOU'RE THE PATIENT

PART II:
WHEN YOU'RE "THOSE WHO LOVE THEM"

ACKNOWLEDGMENTS

I want to thank all the good folks at the Carle Cancer Center in Urbana, Illinois, who worked to get me well, especially my oncologist, Alan Hatfield, and all my nurses, the pharmacists, the social workers, and the front desk personnel. Becky, Evelyn, Sarah, Olivia, Barry, Toni, Judy, Linda, Joni, Laura, Melissa, Nancy, Ron, Joan, Jill, Sharon, Pam, Debbi, I hope you know how important you are to those of us who love you so much but never want to see you again!

Special thanks go to all the members of the Carle Cancer Center support group, especially our social worker and friend, Jeanette Pritschet. I was supported by them, and I learned so much from them.

I also learned from my classmates in "Empowering the Cancer Patient" at Iliff Seminary in Denver. John Anduri, the late Paul K. Hamilton, M.D., and Lynn Ringer, the leaders of that group, have made wholeness in the midst of cancer possible not only for Helen and me but for thousands of other cancer patients. Their story is told in *I'm a Patient, Too,* by Albert Hill.

Paul and Lynn founded CanSurmount. In introducing me at CanSurmount's twentieth anniversary celebration in Denver, Paul did me the honor of calling *Now That I Have Cancer, I Am Whole* "the best book by a cancer patient, for cancer patients, ever."

Fellow patients Jean Cramer-Heuerman, Nancy Nichols, and Kim Wagler Ziner read some of these meditations while the thoughts were still in the hatching stage, and I thank them for their kindness.

Kim Wagler was my first cancer nurse. Hardly a year had gone by after she initiated me into the mysteries of chemotherapy and how to deal with it than she became a cancer patient, too. She is precious to me not only as my nurse but as a fellow traveler in the cancer journey.

Helen says I must have some sort of record for a cancer patient who performs weddings for his nurses, having done so for both Kim and Becky Elliott. Becky usually wore a white uniform dress in the chemo room. Because she always made me throw up (see the meditation "I get sick when I see Becky," page 64), when she asked me to officiate at her wedding, I said, "Don't wear a white dress!" She said her pearls would protect her. After the wedding, she thanked me for not throwing up on her, and I thanked her for keeping me alive, and we had a good time crying on each other.

Rose Mary Shepherd and Rachael Grace Richardson have been guides and models in the cancer walk. Sharon Butts has walked it with me, even though she's never had it. Thank you.

I have been formed by a large, extended family of Ponds and McFarlands. They gave me a sense of belonging. Most important in that sense of belonging, of course, were my parents, John Francis and Mildred Elizabeth, my sisters, Mary Virginia and Margaret Ann, and my brother, James Francis. And no one in the family will ever forget the remarkable Henrietta Ann, "Grandma Mac."

Grandparenting looked like so much fun that early in our marriage, Helen and I contemplated adopting grown-up children so we could go directly to grandchildren. We're glad we didn't, but we're also glad we finally got to the stage of Biddey and Joey.

I have been supported through my cancer journey by more people in more churches than I can possibly name. Especially important to me are those of the Forsythe United Methodist Church (UMC), near Oakland City, Indiana, and those of the Arcola, Illinois, UMC. The good folks at Forsythe accepted me and loved me as a child and teenager. The family of the Arcola UMC kept me going through the difficult days of recovery from surgery and chemotherapy. Moreover, they let me minister to them by getting well in front of them. For that, I'll be forever grateful.

When Joseph was diagnosed with hepatoblastoma when he was only fifteen months old, he spent the next year alternating between Children's Hospital at University Hospital in Iowa City, Iowa, and Mercy Medical Center–North Iowa in Mason City. We thank the doctors and nurses at both hospitals. Chief among them were Dr. Sue O'Dorisio, Joey's personal oncologist, and doctors Jorge Di Paola, Fred Goldman, Thomas Loew, Anthony Sandler, Raymond Tannous, and Rajeev Vibakhar and their assistants, Jane Caswell, Steve Rummelhart, and Mary Schlapkohl. The nurses fought (in a polite way, of course) for the chance to have charge of Joey. Nicole Alcorn usually won. But we could not have made it without the competence and grace of Amy, Beth, Dan, Dom, Gail, Jill, Laurie, Mary Lou, Richard, Rose, and Tom. The Child Life folks (Brenda, Gwen, Jenny, Joie, Kathy, and Robin) provided distraction for Joey and the other children, and relief for the parents, with music and play. Ed Zastrow, Kelly Lamb, and Robyn Welk provided hospitality at the Ronald McDonald House. I'm sure I've omitted many others, but it's absence of memory, not lack of appreciation. Thanks to all who got us through the time when the worst thing possible happened.

Everyone should have friends like George and Ida Belle Paterson. They were parents and grandparents in residence in Iowa City when Helen and I could not be there and gracious hosts to us when we could be.

We thank our friends at Wesley UMC in Mason City for keeping us going while Joey was in the hospital and Brigid lived so much of the time at our house. Bill and Judy Poland, Joyce Hopp, and so many others at Wesley were the neighbors and friends you dream of having all the time.

Our older daughter, Mary Beth, appears in these pages as a cancer survivor herself. While I recovered from rotator cuff surgery, she took over preparing the manuscript in her usual pleasant and efficient manner. Thanks, Bethey.

Thanks once again to the folks at Andrews McMeel. The first edition got into print because of Donna Martin, Patty Donnelly, Dorothy O'Brien, Jean Lowe, Kathy Viele, and Matt Lombardi. It got onto tape because of Anne Gaudinier, Rick Harris, and Rich Romaniano at HarperAudio. The beautiful cover was designed by George Diggs. The revised edition is in your hands because of Christine Schillig, Lane Butler, and Carol Anne Peschke.

The poem "Endangered Species" originally appeared in the April 1991 edition of *The Midwest Poetry Review*.

"Stealing Donkeys" appeared in a slightly different form in *The Christian Century* of March 18, 1990. The poem "Pain" appeared in the same publication for November 14, 1990.

INTRODUCTION

N ot long ago, a woman called our house. My wife answered. Someone had recommended the first edition of this book to her, the woman said, but before she committed herself to buying a copy, she wanted to learn whether I were still alive. Helen was happy to tell her she could go ahead and buy the book.

I'm still here, and the book is back. But my cancer story is longer, and so is the book.

February 1990 started me on a journey of surgery, twelve months of chemotherapy, and two years of fear and healing that produced the 1993 edition of this book.

When I finished the manuscript for the first edition, the subtitle was only *Meditations for Cancer Patients.* I had written primarily as a patient for other patients. But then I added *And Those Who Love Them* because I thought friends and family members could profit from reading how we patients feel.

I certainly did not expect to move from the first category, *Cancer Patients,* to the second category, *Those Who Love Them.* Just as I did not expect to become a patient myself, I did not expect to become the son, brother, husband, father, and grandfather of cancer patients. But that has been my journey over the last dozen years.

It all started with my own cancer, which was a total surprise. Half of health depends on your genes, and I was secure in that half. Before me there had been only two people with cancer among the two hundred relatives in four generations of McFarlands and Ponds. Both of them were well past their eightieth birthday at the first sign.

The other half of health is lifestyle, and I was okay there, too. My meals were prepared by a professional home economist, my wife. I was a long-distance runner and a third baseman. I received a lot of satisfaction from my work and a lot of love from my family and friends.

Nothing to be concerned about, right? Besides, I had no symptoms of any kind. I was almost arrogant in my health until a midnight pain "down south," on my birthday, caused the surgeon to wheel me into the operating room at midnight to have a look. He ended up cutting out a third of my colon and a malignant tumor.

A few days later, my first oncologist said, "You've got it." I had no idea what "it" was. Cancer had never occurred to me, not even as I went to surgery. Careless words from that oncologist hit me as a death sentence. I would be dead "in one to two years."

I was thrown for a loop. My life was turned upside down. The change was so complete that I started every sentence with "Now that I have cancer," a phrase that marked off my present days from all that had gone before. My friend Bill White, who appears in the "It's a touching time" meditation, must have gotten tired of hearing it, because he said, "That sounds like the title of a book." So it is.

It started out as a cancer journal. I read that the recovery rate for cancer patients who put down their thoughts and feelings in a journal is much better than for those who don't. I wasn't about to pass up an opportunity like that.

As I wrote, I realized it wasn't just a journal. I was on a journey, although I wasn't sure of the destination. I came to understand that many others are on that same journey, with similar doubts about where it will lead and where it will end. I became less and less satisfied with simply recording my own expedition. I knew I needed to say a word to and for the others who share the cancer walk. These are my reflections, but they are not mine alone. I like to think of this as a common journal for all of us who must make this trip.

So this book is in part the story of my own cancer journey and those who support me in it. It is also the story of the journeys of others, who have honored me by letting me walk a way with them and learn from them. Most importantly, it is a way of sharing the journey. We know you've got to walk that lonesome valley by yourself. We also know, paradoxically, that we need company on that trip. We're alone and yet together, what my friend Linda Zimmermann once called "a sense of shared privacy."

I have written each meditation from my own experience rather than in a generalized fashion because cancer is a very individual disease. We are not statistics, percentages, or categories; we are people. Cancer is an equal-opportunity disease, however. It strikes rich and poor, young and old, good and bad, red and yellow, black and white. In that way we all share the same road. I trust that in these meditations you will see your own story as I share mine.

We are on a journey, but it is a trip of individual steps. We need to live in the moment, and sometimes that's all we can do. We get by one day at a time, and often only one minute at a time. It's sometimes difficult for us even to hold a big book, let alone read one. We concentrate best in short bursts, on one idea at a time. It is hard to sort through many pages and long chapters, raw knowledge and strange new terms, to find the words we need to hear in our particular moment of need.

So this book is divided into categories that we cancer people understand: steps of the journey. There is no beginning and no end. Feel free to read the meditations in whatever order is best for you, according to which step you're taking at the moment.

The life change that cancer forces is so huge, so overwhelming, especially if surgery, chemotherapy, or radiation adds another misery to the mix. It's hard to get hold of, like trying to play catch with a watermelon when you're used to a baseball. So we tend to pick up on the little changes and events of cancer. It's easier to talk about making offerings to the big white god or how we'll look in a wig than to consider whether chemo will actually move us toward a cure.

That's good. We live in stories, not in abstract theories. Dealing with strange bras and stuck eyelids and bald heads will lead us on to the wider and deeper issues easily enough. The little changes break open the potential for meaning, like the little change in an eggshell at a chick's first peck. So these meditations usually start with some mundane observation or event, such as getting sick when I see Becky, my chemo pusher, even if I see her at a theater. They start there because those are the events of our cancer journey. What they mean . . . well, we can consider that as we walk along together.

It was on my birthday that they cut me open and found the cancer. It was on Helen's birthday that I began a year of chemotherapy. My veins started breaking down from the chemo, so I had to get a Groshong catheter in my chest to save the veins. (They use ports now.) They installed that on our wedding anniversary, of course. We began to dread special days. We came to understand, though, that even with—and perhaps especially with—cancer, every day is a special day.

It was on those everyday special days that I wrote these meditations. I have left them as they were then, when I first heard "that word," when the chemotherapy made me "call Ralph on the big white phone," when I wondered what I'd done to cause this, when I was sick and tired of being sick and tired.

My chemo is long past. I feel good. I'm officially cured. There's a temptation to go back and rewrite the meditations of the early days and the chemo days and the down days, to give them the benefit of the long view. I've not yielded to that temptation, though. At each of those steps, the way it is is the way it is. When you're there, you're there. That's okay.

The story did not end with my own cancer. It continued with my father, and then my mother, and then my brother, Jim, and my grandson, Joseph, and my wife, and my daughter, Mary Beth, and now my little sister, Margey. The meditations I wrote as part of their journey, as one of *Those Who Love Them,* are in Part II of this book. Like those in Part I, they are just as raw as when I wrote them because when you're there, you're there, and that's okay.

PART I
WHEN YOU'RE THE PATIENT

1. WHEN YOU FIRST HEAR "THAT WORD"

(DIAGNOSIS)

Now that I have cancer . . .

. . . *I say "that word" all the time.*

CANCER! THERE. I DID IT.

Some folks are actually afraid of the word itself, aren't they? Have you noticed? They refer to your "trouble," or your "disease," or your "struggle." They just can't bring themselves to say CANCER.

I understand how they feel. I'm more than a little bit afraid of CANCER myself. That's why I say it every time I get the chance. CANCER.

People are afraid to speak that word because they know that words have power. Tell a child often enough that he's stupid, and he'll believe it. Tell her that she's bright, and she'll believe that, too.

My friend Jim McKnight once asked me why our children turned out so well. I can't understand why he seemed surprised that my kids weren't odd. I told him that it was simple: We just gave them everything they wanted and bragged on them all the time. (Our children tell a somewhat different version.) I firmly believe there will be enough people in life who will cut your children down that they don't need it from their parents, too. Brag on them; those words have power.

I know of a church on a university campus that was having trouble keeping its grass alive. The students were cutting across the churchyard on their way to class and wearing a huge path in it. They put up a sign that said "Keep off the grass." It did no good at all. Then, however, they changed the sign to "Let it live." The students used the sidewalk. The right word is a lever that can move the world.

When I was little, my mother taught me a little epigram to use against the neighborhood bullies: "Sticks and stones may break my bones, but words will never hurt me." It would have worked

4

better if the bullies hadn't used sticks and stones as well as words. They certainly knew how to use words, though, and those hurt more than the sticks and stones. It's infuriating to be called "yellow" by three boys who are twice as big as you are. You know that they are the true cowards because they have to gang together and pick on someone smaller. As a child, however, you can't even find the right words so you can tell them that. You just run away.

CBS news reporter Bob Simon was a prisoner of the Iraqis for several weeks in 1991, during the first Persian Gulf War. He said that the words were worse than the beatings. "After a while," he said, "you realize that a beating, although unpleasant and painful, will come to a stop. The terror they put into you with words, however, goes on and on."

Sticks and stones can break your bones, but the words of terror break your spirit.

The terror of that word, CANCER, can go on and on if we don't say it. Saying it puts it into the light and takes away so much of its power.

Sure, I'm still afraid. I could say CANCER all day long, and I'd keep on being scared. But when you speak it right out loud, CANCER isn't very strong. It has strength only in the dark. It can break my body. There may even be times when it will break my spirit. But I know that CANCER is weak. It can't break LOVE. There's no way CANCER can take me away from the love of my wife and my children and grandchildren and my family and my friends and God.

Now that I have cancer, I say that word all the time.
You know the one I mean: LOVE.

. . . Cancer is the answer.

THAT'S WHAT A FRIEND told me when she first heard that word. "I've been looking for something all my life. I've tried booze and drugs and whatever else I could think of. I've been depressed for forty years. I prayed to die. Now, cancer is the answer."

I think I know what she meant. As I sat in my hospital bed, invaded by tubes and lost in a cloud of uncertainty, I had the same feeling. Oh, that wasn't all I felt. Anger and fear and despair and lostness and sadness and hope all called for their turn, too. But cancer was an answer. It pulled all the loose threads together. It was the pivot around which everything else whirled, like the post for a game of tetherball. No one, including me, looked for me to deal with anything else at all. That was a feeling of great relief. I could let everything loose, as a snake wiggles out of an old skin. It was all so simple—just cancer and me.

An oncologist's careless words helped that feeling along. I understood from him that I would be dead in a year or two. I would have thought it even had he not spoken the words. In our society, we equate cancer with death. Nothing focuses the mind like a literal deadline. I didn't like what I heard, but there were no distractions to it. Cancer was the answer; all my other concerns and worries were pushed aside, like so many unread newspapers that get tossed into the recycling bin while you're not looking. The deck is cleared.

Unlike my friend, I've rarely been depressed, but I was then. Studies show that a patient's condition deteriorates rapidly right after he or she hears the diagnosis. Depression follows that word as surely as "Wait till next year" follows a Cubs fan. Depression is literally a low place. I wanted to sink down into that low place and stay there.

There's a seductiveness in cancer. It cleared my calendar so nicely. I could get ready to die with a clear conscience, nothing left undone because I couldn't be expected to do anything. There's a perverse comfort in illness. You just lie there, no expectations.

While I was still in the hospital recovering from surgery, an old college friend, Judith Unger, gave me a copy of Bernie Siegel's *Love, Medicine, & Miracles*. In it he asks, "Why do you need the cancer?" In other words, to what is it the answer? My friend says she needs it in order to die, the answer to her prayer. I guess my answer is that I needed to have my life simplified to the point that I got permission to concentrate on the only important thing there is.

Cancer is a very personal disease. We must each answer that question, "Why do you need it?" When we've answered, however, we find it's only the first question in a line that stretches clear over the hill. So I needed it to die, or to get clear of life's baggage, or something else. But what now? How do I deal with it? Do I just curl up and write "The End" to my story? Do I fight it somehow? It's just me and cancer, yes, eyeball to eyeball, like a matador and a bull in the middle of the ring, not even aware of the sun and the dust and the shouts of the crowd. But we still have to deal with each other. Who will blink first?

Cancer is the answer, but it's another question. What's important to me? What's the meaning of life? How do I find love?

Like my friend, we've looked for love in all the wrong places—in booze and dollars and degrees and promotions and sex and power and work and thrills. We've filled our lives with doing. So often our deeds have erased our actual lives, our being. The question now is not "What do I do?" but "Who am I?" We answer cancer not with more activities, although learning and treatment and medication and visualization may be things we need to do.

We answer cancer with love, with simple being, with the knowledge that each life ends as it started: unbidden, naked, without knowledge of what will be. I am. I am, now, in this moment. There is no certainty in this life, only trust.

That's what I tried to say to my friend. Yes, cancer is the answer. You needed it so you could be broken into pieces so small that you can be put back together in ways you've never even thought about. None of us needs death or cancer. They're just ways of telling us that we need love.

When Moses asked God for a name, God simply replied, "I am who I am." That's all there is. It comes to us at sunrise and sunset, in a simple act of kindness, in a gentle human touch, in music that reaches the spirit deep within, in the knowledge that all that ever was and all that ever will be is here, right now, in this moment. We live by grace, not only in general, but moment to moment. Cancer tells me that.

Now that I have cancer, cancer is the answer.

2. WHEN A PART OF YOU IS GONE

(SURGERY AND RECOVERY)

Now that I have cancer . . .

. . . A part of me is gone.

THEY TOOK OUT ONE third of my colon. I've lost it. I'm not whole anymore.

A lot of us are no longer whole. Cancer patients lose breasts and kidneys and thyroids and lungs and sections of livers and about any other body part we can name. In treatment we can also lose hair and bowel control and even our dinner! We're not only unwhole, we're "losers," too.

Think about those common words, *whole* and *loser*. They take on different meanings when we put them in the cancer context, don't they?

Most of the time we can disguise the fact that we aren't whole, that we are losers. We have wigs and turbans and prostheses and body-hugging colostomy bags. They're good things. If you lose your teeth, you get false ones. What's wrong with doing the same thing if you lose breasts or hair? Sure, some of it's just cosmetic, but there's nothing wrong with looking good. Anything we can do to feel better about ourselves, let's do it!

However, even when we're looking our best, we know there's something missing. Some losses can't be replaced. I'll never get another colon.

Jesus had something to say about this. "If your eye or your hand causes you to sin, pluck it out or cut it off and throw it away; it is better that you lose one of your members than that your whole body be thrown into hell. And if your hand causes you to sin, cut it off and throw it away" (Matthew 5:29–30).

(It's very easy to get lost in the trees here and thus not see the forest. Are heaven and hell literal places? Did Jesus mean you should physically cut off your hand? Interesting questions, but they are trees, not the forest.)

Sin breaks relationships. Sin breaks us apart from God and our neighbors and our own true selves. Sin fragments us, makes us unwhole. Sin causes us to lose what is most important in life, the relationships through which love comes.

Ah, there are those words again: *unwhole, loser*.

Jesus is saying that it's not the physical loss that makes us unwhole, that makes us losers. In fact, he says, even if something so physically important as an eye or hand makes us lose that which is most important, love, then it is good to be a loser, good to be unwhole in our physical bodies so that we can be whole in love.

The point Jesus was making (the forest rather than the trees) is that true wholeness has nothing to do with whether our bodies would make good charts for anatomy students. The one who plucks out an eye or cuts off a hand because it is breaking relationships, because it is walling us off from love, is more whole than the one who's never lost a part but uses those parts to hurt.

My friend Max White always says, as he prays in church, "Bless those of us assembled here." It's a marvelous phrase. He means, of course, bless those of us who have come together in this one location from our separate places. The word *assembled* has an individual meaning as well. It refers to each one of us being put together, being made whole. "Bless those of us who are being put together here."

Sin separates us. Coming together in love assembles us, puts us together.

In a strange way, I feel more assembled, more put together, since I've lost a part of my body than I did before. Cancer has brought me closer to God and to those who love me and to my own true self. In that sense, good health was a sin. As long as I could keep going day by day without even thinking about my health, it was also easy for me to take love for granted. Like Scarlett O'Hara, I could think about that tomorrow.

Cancer reminds us that there is no tomorrow, just as there is no yesterday. For love, there is only today.

Now that I have cancer, a part of me is missing.
Ironically, I'm more whole, more a winner of love,
than I've ever been before.

*. . . I am learning to see myself
through the eyes of love.*

THOSE WHO LOVE ME have much better eyes than I. The eyes
of love are always best. Love is not blind at all. Love sees with
the eyes of God, not the eyes of the world. Love has remarkable
clarity of vision, the scope of an eagle, free from all those floating
debris spots of "reality."

There was something about me, before cancer, that I could
not love. Not all of me, but something. I must have hated it so
much, to create a cancer that required my own mutilation, to
demand that a part of me be cut out and thrown away. I don't
quite understand that, but somehow I feel its truth. It's like when
you have set the alarm for six in the morning, and you wake
up just before the bell rings for you, even though you normally
snooze steadily on until seven. The body knows.

You may not feel that way at all. I have a cancer friend who
says, "I'm blameless. I didn't do anything at all to cause this." I
believe her. She knows herself. I know myself, too.

I look at me with the eyes of reality, and what do I see? A
scrawny, hairless man. Those formerly marvelous, marathoning
muscles just hang on bones of unproductive and depleted marrow.
The bright blue eyes are bloodshot. They peek out through tiny
slits where my eyelids have glued themselves to each other. This
skinny man is bent over, divided by an angry, red scar that looks
like an N-gauge model railroad track. The veins beneath my skin
look like jagged and jaded lightning flashes, as if I had gotten
caught in a bleach storm in my Captain Marvel suit. My lips are
red and puffy, like a sad circus clown. That's the view through the
eyes of reality.

Then there are the eyes of love. My wife sighs, "Every time

I look at you, I fall in love all over again." My daughters say, "Remember what good times we had when we were little girls and you lay down on the sofa after supper and we'd sit on the back of it and roll you off with our feet? You're the best dad ever." My teammates call to say, "Hurry back. Nobody else has the reflexes to play third base as close to the batter as you do." A woman tells me, "I'd be dead except for the hope you gave me." A now-grown man says, "You have no idea how important you were to all of us on campus in the sixties. You made us believe we could make a difference." God says, "I love you just the way you are."

Those aren't the eyes of reality; those are the eyes of love. They see me as I want to be and yet, for them, already am.

Now that I have cancer, I can see myself through their eyes. I like seeing me through the eyes of love.

. . . I sing.

I ALWAYS ENJOYED SINGING, but now I sing all the time. It's almost impossible to sing a full-throated note and be tied up by fear at the same time.

I sing all sorts of songs—hymns and ballads and pop and scat and blues and rock and folk and opera—anything that comes to mind. I make up crazy songs as I go along, too. Sometimes the words make sense, sometimes not. Sometimes they rhyme, other times not. Some have familiar tunes, but some of those I make up as well.

One of the most frustrating things for me when I first came home from the hospital was that I couldn't sing. The tube up my nose and down my throat left me sounding like Donald Duck with a cold. I had been cut open from Los Angeles to Boston. Every muscle in my abdomen was spending all its energy just trying to get reconnected. I had no power from my diaphragm. All I could do was mouth the words.

Well, I decided, if that's all I can do, that's what I'll do. Better to sing a wee, tiny song than no song at all.

Like most doors that close, this one caused another to open. Since I couldn't sing very well, I began to compose. "Compose" isn't quite the right word. I began to "adjust" songs.

I sing them in the bathtub mostly. That's probably safest. While I lie in the warm water, Emmett Kelly, the clown, comes and sweeps my body clean with his spotlight broom. (If you've not read the meditation on commitment yet, see page 43 for more about Emmett.) He does each part, each organ, of my body. I sing to help him along. My, how that clown can sweep out cancer cells when he has a little music!

As I wash my hair, I sing, "Gonna wash that cancer right out of myself . . . and send it on its way." I adjusted the spiritual "Oh,

Freedom." I sing, "No more cancer. No more cancer. No more cancer inside of me. And before I'll be a slave, I'll put cancer in its grave, and go home to my Lord, and be free." To the tune of "If You're Happy and You Know It, Clap Your Hands" I sing, "I'm glad I'm a little cake of soap. (Repeat.) I'll slippie and I'll slidie all over my hidie and I'll wash the cancer off with my soap."

Okay, so they're pretty bad, but they're just for Emmett and me, and they work.

I don't mean singing works by automatically wafting cancer away on a tune. It might help, but who knows? I do know that it works by taking away the fear.

You just can't sing and be afraid at the same time. That's why we sing in the dark. It is also very difficult to sing and awfulize at the same time. Awfulizing is the process of imagining all the awful things that might happen to us. We spend more time at it than we realize. The less awfulizing we do, the more likely we are to get well. The immune system doesn't like awfulizing; it does like singing.

Singing is as natural as loving. In fact, they are very closely related—two limbs from one trunk, from one root system. Together they spread out a canopy of shade.

Both those limbs get weather-beaten, however. They are besieged by frost and drought and hail and acid rain and parasites and blight. It's a wonder they survive at all, and in some folks I guess they don't. But their tree is rooted deep in the soil of the Spirit.

With all those blights and plights attacking them, though, what was so natural becomes unnatural. How many people refuse to sing, claim they can't sing, give all sorts of excuses—from illness to shyness—why they mustn't sing? We do the same with loving. We're afraid we'll be hurt. We have already been hurt. We're afraid we'll be rejected or look silly.

I suspect we can learn a lot about how we love by how we sing.

The search for healing and wholeness includes singing. You don't have to go on stage. You don't even have to use a recognizable tune or sing on key. Just croak out whatever words you remember or that come to you. Sing your prayers and sing away your fears. Do it in the bathroom with the water running. Sing along with Johnny Mathis or Dolly Parton or Mick Jagger.

Singing leaves no room for fear. Even if singing doesn't cure us, it does help to heal us. That, after all, is the goal of life: not just to live a long time but to live well.

Now that I have cancer, I sing. Try it: "Happy days are here again. The cancer's gone away again."

. . . _I do something each day._

IT MAY NOT SOUND like much of a goal, but three weeks after my surgery, "something every day" is a big step forward. Of course, I've been doing the necessities for recovering from surgery and preventing complications: deep breathing, walking the loop from my bedroom to the family room and through the living room and back down the hall again, sleeping ten hours a night plus an afternoon nap, eating a gentle four meals a day. After all those necessaries are done and I've read a few pages of Bernie Siegel or Greg Anderson or Joan Borysenko, something is all I have time and energy for.

By "something," I mean making a telephone call, writing a letter, or doing the dishes. It's not much, is it? I used to run five miles and then work ten or twelve hours without a break. I made a dozen telephone calls and wrote enough letters to make the postal service smile, saw a mob of people, and still got the dishes done and walked the dog. Now Waggs just hangs around the door with drooping tail until Helen notices that it's walk time.

Now, however, my daily something takes more concentration and planning and discipline than all the tasks that used to race through my days put together. I know that if I choose to write one letter, it means I can't write to anyone else. Which letter is most important? Or should I be sure today that Helen finds a clean kitchen when she returns home from a day of dealing with boisterous teenagers? When you have only one thing you can do, how do you decide which one thing it is?

Clear back in the summer of 1964, when Henry Aaron was playing for the Milwaukee Braves and John Roseboro was catching for the Dodgers, Aaron came to bat in a game between the two teams. Roseboro noticed that Aaron had the brand of the bat to the front, toward the pitcher. The brand is the place where the information about the bat—the name of the manufacturer and so on—is burned into the wood. Every sandlot baseball player knows you always bat with the brand to the back because the bat is likely to break if it and the ball connect directly on the brand.

"Hey, you've got the brand to the front," said Roseboro.

Aaron looked at it, left it where it was, took his stance, and said, "I didn't come up here to read."

It's no surprise that Hank Aaron is the all-time leading home run hitter. He knew what his one something was: He was up there to hit.

It's important to concentrate on the one something I have to do, to experience it rather than just do it, to concentrate on it and feel it rather than just marking it off a list so I can go on to something else.

As I come to bat, it's tempting to say the one thing I'm up here for is to get well, to hit the long ball, to take cancer over the wall and out of the park. I'd like that. The homer, though, is simply the end product of many little somethings: the openness of the stance, the tilt of the bat, the keenness of eye to see whether the pitch is in the strike zone, the shift of the weight, the snap of the wrists. All those little somethings put together were what made Aaron the homer champ.

My turn at bat isn't just to get well but to do well, to concentrate on each event of the day, to pay attention to the little things, because the only way I have to love is in that one swing. My something each day now is more important than all the masses of things I used to do. Whether I live long or short, in pain or without pain, I have one thing to do each day, regardless of how many ways that one thing may be expressed. Into each letter, each phone call, each washed dish, I put the full measure of all my love. I think by doing well, I'm helping myself get well, but that's not the point. Søren Kierkegaard wrote, "Purity of heart is to will one thing." Whether it's a home run or a sacrifice bunt, my turn at bat is to do one thing: to love.

Now that I have cancer, I do something each day.

. . . *I'm learning to live with limits.*

NOT THAT I DIDN'T have limits before. Before, though, my limits
were pretty far out. I knew I'd never play first base for the Reds,
run a marathon under three hours, or be asked to a dinner party at
Sophia Loren's house. But I could play third base for "The Fossils"
in the Rocking Chair League. I could run a marathon under four
hours. I was asked to dinner parties at Pat Meyerholtz's house.
Maybe I'll play softball with the old guys again sometime. Maybe
I'll even run a marathon again, when the chemo is over and the
Groshong catheter is out of my chest and I'm not tired so much
of the time. Pat and Roy still invite me to their house, as do other
friends. When the cold and flu season is over and my immune
system is no longer depressed, maybe I'll be able to enjoy those
homemade rolls and that home-style friendship once more.

In the meantime, I can't go to ball games, or restaurants, or
other places where people and germs gather. I can't do anything
where I'll get cut because the Coumadin has thinned my blood
and I won't heal very well. Helen has to crawl under the house
to adjust the vents as the seasons change. John Mills cleans my
gutters. Bill Alexander mows my yard. Ross and Paulina Hunt
weed my flowers. Sometimes I feel pretty helpless. This I know,
though: Every new limitation is a new challenge. When my body
was young and supple, I could do with it whatever I wanted to,
almost. Now, suddenly, all these restrictions. However, they are
the restrictions that lead to creativity.

If Beethoven had not lived within the restrictions that musical
form imposes, the creativity that produced those wonderful
symphonies would never have been possible. If you don't believe
me, just listen to some of the undisciplined "music" that surrounds
us today. It is not creative because it is not first disciplined. Ted

Williams, Joe Morgan, and the other great baseball hitters were successful because they disciplined themselves to know when a pitch was in the strike zone, when it was a fastball and when a curve. They didn't swing at the pitches they knew they couldn't hit, so they hit more than most. They lived within their limitations, and they were successful.

Okay, the restrictions of cancer are not always pleasant or desirable. But they can lead to creativity. You have to learn new ways of doing, of being, of getting things done. If you can't get the old things done, you have to learn new things to do. If I could be out playing third base or running marathons or talking with my friends, I wouldn't be writing these words.

One of the gifts of cancer is the challenge, the challenge to live within new limitations, to have our lives renewed at the very moment we are dis-eased. After all, that is what a challenge is, being at dis-ease with what has been, so that something new can take its place.

Harry Houdini, the great escape artist, used to say, "The smaller the box, the greater the escape."

I'm learning what it is to have a part of my body burned out to make room for the spirit to grow.

Now that I have cancer, I'm learning to live with limits.

. . . I make sure I know where I am.

NO ONE ELSE DOES.

That's overstating the case a bit. My wife and children know where I am. Many of my friends do. The dog always does when she wants a snack. I'm sure God does.

But my doctor didn't. The day after my operation, my surgeon went on vacation. That's fine; I like for surgeons to be well rested. His partner came to see me while he was out of town. When he returned to the hospital, however, the partner stopped coming. My doctor didn't show up, either.

I was supposed to be moving from clear liquids to full liquids to a solid diet, but they had me stuck on the clear stuff. You know, the grape juice they strain through nuclear waste to give it that special taste. I was getting light-headed and nauseous from lack of food, but the nurses said they couldn't move me up on the food chain because the doctors had written no new orders. Finally, when I got that story one night at about 8:30, I wailed, "But the doctors couldn't write any new orders. They haven't been in for three days."

"Three days? Are you sure?"

It was actually only about two and a half, but for the first time since I was wheeled into the hospital, I sensed I had the serve. I wasn't going to lose it over twelve hours of night.

"Yes, three," I said. "Maybe they died. Maybe their AA meeting ran long. Maybe they moved and didn't tell anyone. Aren't they required to give two weeks' notice if they quit?"

I was enjoying this. I was on a roll. So was Paula, the night nurse. It was a delight to see her hustle out of the room to phone those doctors. All of a sudden I realized it: I had control!

She returned and said, "The kitchen is closed, but they said you can have whatever we've got, which is ice cream and graham crackers."

23

"You mean I can go straight from that awful grape juice to ice cream?"

"They said you can try anything. If you keep it down, you can go home. I think they feel a little guilty. Your surgeon forgot you were here."

That ice cream just about gagged me, but I shambled through the halls all night, willing it to stay where it was. It did. I went home.

He forgot I was there! My own surgeon, who rightly has a reputation as one of the best around, who knows my insides more intimately than anyone but God, forgot I was in the hospital! He didn't know I was there.

I thought all I had to do was lie there, and someone would take care of me. It wouldn't take any thought or action from me at all. Not so, I found. It's my life. I've got to take care of it. I'm the only one who really knows where I am.

I guess I am in the middle 70 percent that has to be taught to take control of our own lives. There is a 15 percent group that does it automatically. They're the aggressive type; it's a good type to be when you are sick. There is another 15 percent that just rolls over and dies, regardless of what anyone tries to do for them. We middle 70 percent can take control, can be responsible for ourselves, but we have to learn to do it.

Now I thank God that my surgeon forgot where I was. His forgetfulness gave me a great gift, the gift of control, the responsibility for my own wellness.

We can't just sit back and expect someone else to do it. Sure, we all need help. I couldn't have operated on myself. I couldn't prescribe chemo for myself. There are days I can't do anything by myself. But I am the one who has to know where I am, and where I want to be. Otherwise, I won't be there.

Now that I have cancer, I make sure I know where I am.

. . . I'm in a prison of pain.

I CAN'T COMMUNICATE ABOUT it, and I can't admit anyone else into it. Others cannot get into my cell even if they want to. The pain is a wall between us. We might as well be in separate worlds.

The rule of ninety and ten applies. In major surgery, the patient's life is changed 90 percent. The patient retains only 10 percent contact with his former life. Those around him are changed only 10 percent by the surgery; they retain 90 percent of their former lives—jobs, household chores, regular routines.

I can interact only with and to pain and to 10 percent of the life of those around me. Therefore, they end up ignoring me and relating to one another because it is more natural for them; they still share 90 percent with one another, only 10 percent with me. They talk about me. They talk to one another. Rarely do they talk to me.

So I have become a management problem rather than a person—to the hospital, to my family, to visitors. They see me in my pain and don't know what to do about it. They've never seen me this way before. I understand, but it hurts—not just the pain, but not being a person.

When we are sick, we are overwhelmed by the illness. It becomes our only reality. It's not that we have a clear focus and thus don't see the rest of the world around us, like an athlete who shuts out the crowd noise as she concentrates on the point where the racket smacks the ball. It's more like being in a thick fog, so that we have no focus at all. When you are in pain, the pain takes over. You can't think about anything else. You can't think at all; you can only feel.

I believe that's why we get so spiritual at times like this, so "religious," if you will. I know I've "gotten religion," which is an especially ironic thing for me to say since I've spent my adult life being religious as a profession. But it's like Peter O'Toole's protest

25

in the film *My Favorite Year,* when his character learned he would have to go on live: "But I'm not an actor; I'm a movie star!" When it comes to facing pain, none of us is anything but an amateur.

Thinking is about beliefs, doctrines, ideas—things of the head. Feeling is about pain and joy—things of the heart. Feeling is spiritual; it digs deep into the heart of a truth that cannot be spoken but only experienced. When you are in pain—the pain of surgery and cancer and being a problem instead of a person—thinking drops off and feeling takes over.

Feeling also makes us individuals, just as pain does. No one can share the pain. Nor can anyone tell us how to feel, what is right or wrong to feel. We simply feel whatever we feel, that's all there is to it, be it despair or elation, pain or joy, fear or faith.

It is strange how pain makes us more individual. We are actually more reliant on others physically. We need their care for our bodies, their pain pills and wet cloths. But we have to become more reliant on ourselves spiritually. At the very time others are treating us more as nonpersons because we no longer share their world, at least during the time of our pain, we actually become more real as persons because we are more individual, spiritual, unique.

However, we are so used to thinking instead of feeling that it is hard for us to accept this. Our brains use up all their energy on pain, so we assume nothing significant can come of it. Most of the time we don't even know how we feel. That's why pain takes us over so completely: It requires us to feel instead of to think. It requires us to be spiritual persons instead of social persons.

Now that I have cancer, I'm in a prison of pain. That is also a cell of uniqueness, of feeling, of spirituality. I'm released from thought to walk in the fog and feel its soft and shifting contact. I am a unique person because the pain I feel is mine alone.

26

3. WHEN IT'S

TIME TO FIGHT

(GEARING UP)

Now that I have cancer . . .

. . . It's "no more Mr. Nice Guy."

I DON'T WANT TO be well adjusted to the diagnosis, to my cancer. I don't want to be a "good patient." I don't want my doctor and the chemo nurses and whomever else I deal with to think I'm "nice" and "cooperative." I don't want to be a pain, but I don't want to have a pain, either. The well adjusted don't survive.

The problem is, I don't know how to be anything but nice. I've always been nice. I learned early that you get rewarded for being nice, or at least that you stay out of trouble that way.

I heard a story of a court case. An Amish farmer was suing for damages. It seems a car had collided with his buggy. The judge asked him why he was suing because he had told the investigating police officer at the time of the accident that he wasn't hurt.

"Well," said the farmer, "he went over to my horse. He said, 'This horse is hurt,' and he shot it. Then he went over to my dog. He said, 'This dog is hurt,' and he shot it. Then he came over to me and said, 'Are you hurt?' and I said, 'No, sir!'"

It makes good sense, doesn't it? If you think someone is going to shoot you if you show any hurt, any vulnerability, then you keep saying, "No, sir! Nothing wrong with me." But there are things wrong. There are real hurts in our lives, and they don't get better because we keep them out of sight.

There's a line in the song "Sixteen Tons" that says "Trouble and fightin' are my middle name." I admire that ornery coal miner. I wish "trouble and fightin'" were my middle name. Instead, my middle name is "suppression and fear." (I'll never get a country-western song written about me if I can't get a more lyrical middle name than that.)

What's your middle name? I'll bet it's something like mine, because cancer patients are notorious emotion suppressers.

We're like the man who caught the porcupine under a tub. You've got a darn mad porcupine under there, and no idea which way it'll come out if you don't hold it down. So you just keep sitting on the tub.

Most of us cancer patients get so many porcupines down inside, the really prickly kind, usually without even knowing it. The porcupines don't have any place to go, so they get together and build a tumor just to have a place to hang out.

The tumor gets cut out, or radiated, or flushed out with chemicals, but that doesn't solve the porcupine problem. That just gets rid of the hangout. They'll build another one if we still try to keep them under the tub, if we don't let them leave.

I'm doing better with the porcupine problem. I cry more now. I laugh more, too. If people ask me how I feel, and I feel rotten that day, I don't smile and say, "Oh, just fine." I tell them I feel rotten. (One of the reasons I laugh more now is the expressions on their faces when I tell it like it is.) I see a psychologist; I read that cancer patients who do that have twice as good a survival rate. I'm learning to be honest with her about how I really feel. In fact, I'm learning to be honest with myself.

Every once in a while, I pull up a porcupine that blinks and says, "Whee! Why didn't you let me out of there before?" We both feel better when it's gone.

So look out, world. No more Mr. Nice Guy here. Now that I have cancer, my middle name is "getting sort of honest." It's still not good enough for a song, but keep listening to your radio.

Now that I have cancer, it's "no more Mr. Nice Guy."

. . . I believe in old clichés.

FORMERLY I SCORNED THEM. "When the going gets tough, the tough get going." "Today is the first day of the rest of your life." "I have cancer, but cancer doesn't have me." "No day is over if it makes a memory." "Not everyone will be cured, but everyone can be healed." "There's no problem so great that God and I together can't solve it." "Your disability is your opportunity."

To the uninitiated, they sound like so many bumper stickers. You can't help but be a little cynical about people who live by such simplistic slogans, can you?

My cancer friend, Jean Cramer-Heuerman, whose wisdom and insight appear often in these meditations, used to sit beside me at meetings. Together we laughed behind our hands when someone pulled out one of the old chestnuts. We preferred long and complicated arguments that acknowledged the intricacies that really do inhabit every human situation. (See, you can tell by that sentence.) If we had a slogan, it was Oliver Wendell Holmes's statement, "I'd give anything for the simplicity on the far side of complexity, but nothing for the simplicity on the near side of complexity." Now, even that one takes on new meaning.

Then Jean and I got cancer at about the same time. She says that when you get cancer, suddenly there is new life in the old clichés. It's a form of emotional recycling.

What does it take to deal with cancer? The experts tell us the answer is in four words: three *C*s and an *S*.

The first *C* is *challenge.* You have to accept the challenge cancer gives. In other words, "When the going gets tough, the tough get going." "There's no problem so great that God and I together can't solve it." "Your disability is your opportunity."

The second *C* is *control.* You can't just think of yourself as a victim. In other words, "I have cancer, but cancer doesn't have me." "No day is over if it makes a memory." "Cancer is not a sentence, just a word."

The third *C* is *commitment,* or involvement: "Today is the first day of the rest of your life." "Not everyone will be cured, but everyone can be healed." "I believe." "Be patient with me; God isn't finished yet."

The *S* is *support:* "Jesus loves me, this I know, for the Bible tells me so." "I get by with a little help from my friends." "God made me, and God doesn't make junk."

Well, there you have it. Simple, isn't it? Just take cancer, stir in some old clichés, and you have a recipe for getting by, "one day at a time."

What's your favorite?

Now that I have cancer, I believe in the old clichés.
When you have cancer, they are not clichés anymore,
though, are they?

. . . Baseball is my favorite game.

MAYBE IT ALWAYS WAS. For an old guy, I still have great reflexes. I even stand in front of the mirror every day to admire my reflexes. I play the closest third base of any "hot corner" fielder in the Rocking Chair League. I've got the reflexes and the guts. (I've also got such a weak arm that I have to be halfway to first base when I field a ball or I can't peg it over there.) Being a little stupid doesn't hurt any, either, if you're going to play that close.

I love basketball, too, almost as much as I love chocolate-covered graham crackers. Football is fun, if you like to see big people playing king of the hill without a hill. I get a kick out of soccer. But baseball is definitely my favorite now because time never runs out as long as you have left even one swing at the ball.

The trouble with basketball, football, soccer, and most other games is that they have time limits. When the sixty minutes or the forty minutes have ticked off, that mournful whistle blows. The game is over.

Take football. Football coaches are like oncologists who think they are realists. They pace the sidelines and say, "Only five more minutes." When the game goes into overtime, the loser is subject to "sudden death." Who wants to watch football and cancer at the same time?

But baseball! As the great baseball philosopher Yogi Berra once said, "It ain't over till it's over." Most people think Yogi's dike has a leak when he makes statements like that. You see, though, Yogi is thinking with a baseball mentality. It ain't over when the time runs out. It's only over when the last out is made. You can be down nineteen to one, but as long as you have one more swing, you know you can win. Bottom of the ninth, two out, two strikes on you, down nineteen runs, and you know it ain't over yet!

I come from a long line of baseball players and Cincinnati Reds fans. My great-uncle, Rufus McFarland, played as a boy in Oakland City, Indiana, with Edd Roush, the Reds Hall of Famer. Edd's twin brother, Fred, was one of my coaches when I was a kid, and Edd sometimes came out to the field to hit line drives to us. Uncle Rufus and Edd went up the minors together. A left-side infielder at five feet, three inches, Uncle Rufus figured he would be the shortest man ever to play in the major leagues. Unfortunately, no one wanted a shortstop who really was.

That's a great heritage for a cancer patient. When I'm feeling down, I just play a little baseball. Uncle Rufus and Edd Roush and Pete Rose and Joe Morgan and Johnny Bench—all on my side, you bet! We come to bat in the bottom of the ninth and start swinging. You should see the looks of despair on the faces of the cancer team! They know, as surely as we do, that it ain't over till it's over. In fact, we know it ain't over even when it's over.

Thank you, Yogi. We're up.

Now that I have cancer, baseball is my favorite game.

. . . *I'm accepting the challenge.*

IF YOU'VE READ THE meditation on learning to live with limits, you've already heard me say that I think the challenge cancer brings is one of its gifts. Any gift is just an offer until it is accepted, however. Then it becomes a gift. To be healed, we have to accept the gift of challenge.

Some people have no trouble with that at all. They're always ready for a fight. They have to win regardless of the cost. That's not a bad attitude when cancer comes. Cancer throws down the gauntlet, and the competitors snatch it up before it hits the ground.

Some folks give in and give up as quickly as the competitors jump into the fray. They hear the word *cancer* and just roll over. "What's the use?" they say. "Nothing I can do will make a difference." (If you think you're in this group, take a look at the meditation titled "Cancer is the answer" on page 6. If you've already read it, it's okay to read it again.)

Most of us are confused, though. We don't know what to do or how to do it. Fortunately, when the fog of confusion clears a little, we can be taught. We just have to learn that it's all right to accept the challenge.

I've had to learn. I like to compete in games, but cancer's not a game. I'm not an automatic fighter, but I'm learning to take the challenge. Cancer says, "I'm betting you won't fight." I'm saying back, "In your face! You've got a battle now."

That's what cancer is: a challenge, a slap in the face with a white glove, a summons to a duel. Cancer has done the slapping. Now, according to the ancient rules of duels, we get to choose the weapons.

So I choose: chemotherapy at close quarters, laser swords

(radiation) at three feet, my hope against cancer's fear, my family and friends and nurses and physicians against cancer's sneaky doubts, the God of the Eternal Present against cancer's claim that death ends time, love against cancer's destruction.

One of the marks of a long-term survivor is a sense of purpose in life, a new meaning for life—not in spite of the disease but because of it. Facing down cancer is itself a reason to live.

In one way, of course, a challenge is just an opportunity to fail. What if I accept the challenge but lose the battle? Well, I figure there's no way that can happen, because the victory comes simply in taking the challenge, in not backing down. Here's a little poem:

Love and I
looked death in the eye.
Death blinked.

That's what always happens. Cancer and death are hollow blusterers. They have power only to cause pain and rot to the body. They can't even touch love. The challenge is to choose love, to choose spirit, instead of giving in to fear. When we seize the challenge and shake it by the throat, we have already won.

Tom Dooley, the young medical doctor who worked in Laos in the 1950s, had a dream while in the hospital for cancer treatments. "The mountain in my dream was burned, and now they were planting the new life into the near-dead soil. There was no more self-sadness, no darkness deep inside: no gritty annoyance at anyone or anything. No anger at God for my cancer, no hostility to anyone. I was out of the fog of confusion—standing under the clear light of duty."

Here was a man who knew he was going to die, that his days were numbered on the hands. Still, he accepted the challenge of what that meant. Such a person can never be a failure.

Frankly, if I were cancer, I'd be quaking in my boots. Old

cancer picked the wrong target this time! I'm going to beat this blunderer whether I live or whether I die, because love is on my side. The only allies cancer has are doubt and fear. They don't have a chance.

Now that I have cancer, I'm accepting the challenge.

. . . *I get cards.*

PEOPLE SEND ME ALL sorts of cards. Funny cards. Sentimental cards. Religious cards. I like to get the cards, even when I'm so weak my wife has to read them to me. Even when my hands are so swollen and sore from chemo that I can't open them myself.

Helen taped them to the wall in my hospital room, down at the foot of the bed, where I could see them. One was huge, twelve inches by twenty-four inches. It showed a frightening nurse with a huge needle coming right toward me. I left it there because she made the real nurses and the real needles look so much better. More importantly, that wall reminded me that I had a world outside of the hospital, a world of people who prayed for me and really cared what happened to me.

My first hospital roommate kept a chain saw in bed with him. All night long he tried to start it, without success. My wife claimed he was snoring, but I still hold to the chain saw theory. When he jerked an especially explosive pull on the rope and almost got it going, I would wake up. In the dim light from the hallway I could see my cards on the wall. Even at three in the morning, those cards reminded me that someone, somewhere, in another time zone or aroused by another chain saw (or maybe the same one), was awake and praying for me.

I think the card itself is a prayer, whether the sender means it that way or not. A card says to the sick person, "I care." After all, a prayer is just a way of saying to the universe, "I care."

We can say that in various ways to the sick person, sometimes with words, sometimes with actions. People do things for me: bring me flowers or books, come and spend some time with me, relieve my wife so she can go out for a while, fill in for me on the job, take me to a chemo treatment. Somehow, though, that

37

doesn't seem enough for one we love. There aren't enough of those little tasks to go around, anyway. We grope about for some greater way to reach out with some of our own strength, our own wholeness, our own health to the one who's sick. We shout toward the sky, "I care about what happens to this person!"

Someone has said that when we stand before the judgment seat, the question we'll be asked is not "Did you believe?" but "Did you care?" That's why even nonbelievers pray for those they love.

Prayer isn't telling God or anyone else what to do or how to do it. None of us is smart enough for that.

Monica of ancient Hippo was a religious woman. Her son, Augustine, wanted to go to Rome, because he was a playboy and interested only in his own pleasure. Rome was a happening place. Monica prayed and prayed that her son would not be allowed to make his way to the fleshpots of Rome, for she was sure he would be ruined there. Augustine went anyway. There he heard Ambrose preach, and he was converted. The playboy became the saint.

Was Monica's prayer answered? No, not if you mean getting that for which she prayed. But her real prayer was answered. She had cried out, "I care about this boy," and God answered, "So do I."

With either a card or a prayer, it is difficult to know just what to say. What are the right words *to* one who is sick? We're not sure, so we get a card to say it for us. What are the right words *for* one who is sick, to say to God, to shout to the universe? We're not sure about that, either, so we intone or mumble or cry out our prayers—some comical, some religious, some sentimental, just like cards.

The cards and the prayers both say, "I care."

I have so many cards that if I set them on fire, they'd keep me warm the rest of my life. That's true with prayers, too. I'm blessed and supported by those who pray for me. I can feel those "spirit cards" in my soul.

They say that to get well you need three *C* words and one *S* word: *commitment, challenge, control,* and *support.* Maybe the *S* is a *C,* also: *caring.*

Now that I have cancer, I get cards.

. . . *I'm in control.*

I'M IN CONTROL OF my life, more than I've ever been before.

Sounds strange, doesn't it? You don't have much control of your life when you're a statistic, and I'm definitely a statistic. I'm in that group that has a 70 percent chance of being dead in one to two years. When they put a percentage on you, you're a statistic.

My wife's favorite way of explaining me is to shake her head in what I hope is mock disgust and say, "He's totally out of control." It's the funniest thing, but whenever she says that is when I'm most totally *in* control. I'm in *my* control, singing, laughing, dancing—what *I* want to do, affirming my life.

There are two ways that we get out of control. One is when we lose self-control, when we are driven by forces we don't understand and we can't harness, when we are dragged helplessly behind the wild and raging horses of the emotions. The other is when we break free from the suffocating control that the dead hand of tradition and social expectation wraps around our throat.

In our society, ironically, when we say someone is out of control, we usually mean that person is under self-control, free both from the whirlwind forces on the inside and the brick fences that surround us on the outside.

One of the worst things a sports commentator can say about a ballplayer is that she or he plays out of control. That means that either the player is trying to go beyond the limits of her ability or that he's straying from the coach's game plan.

When it's down to the final minute, however, and the game is on the line, the *best* thing the same commentator can say is that the player stepped up and took control. There is a time when you have to go beyond your own limits, when you have to play above your head, when you dump the game plan and start creating something so unexpected that it will turn defeat into victory. You have to play out of control.

Cancer's like that, I think. The game is there, to be won or lost, now. Those around us still want to control us, even in cancer time. They praise us if we don't complain or admit that we hurt. They want us to be "good patients," which means good victims. They don't want to be bothered or embarrassed by our struggles, by our wild attempts to play out of control. They don't think of it this way, but they'd rather see us lose the game than embarrass ourselves, and them, by trying in some unruly fashion to win.

There's a phrase from sports that's important to us here, though. It's "winning ugly." You look more like Mickey Mouse than Michael Jordan, but you get the ball through the hoop anyway. You swing more like "The Born Loser" than like Ted Williams, but you still get the hit. You don't win pretty, but you win.

I have wondered about a seeming contradiction in the cancer literature I have read. One study shows that patients who participate in volunteer service to others recover better than those who don't. Another study indicates that those most free about saying "no" when asked to do something for others recover better.

I think the contradiction is solved by this matter of control. If one is really a volunteer, working to help others because that is a free choice, then that person has control. On the other hand, if you are coerced or shamed into doing for others, be they family or friends or strangers, the control is taken away from you. We recover better if we have control, regardless of what that means about doing things for others.

To win the cancer battle, along with commitment, challenge, and support, we need control. That means we need both to be in control and to be out of control.

We need to be out of control—out of the control of others, out of the control of our own fears and greed for life. When we're out of control, that's when we're in control.

Now that I have cancer, I'm in control.

. . . *I'm committed.*

THERE ARE PROBABLY THOSE who think I ought to be
"committed," like to an institution, but that's not what I mean.

Support, control, challenge, and commitment, the four
necessities for recovery. Commitment to self-growth and self-
wellness and commitment to something beyond, some greater
growth and greater wellness as well.

Commitment means action, a plan, doing something to get
results. You can be in favor of something but not committed to
it—democracy, for instance. I can say I'm all for democracy, but
if I don't vote, I'm not committed to it. I might think it's a good
idea to help the hungry, but until I give money or volunteer at a
food pantry or lobby my congressman, I'm not really committed
to easing the pangs of hunger.

To resist cancer, I have to take action against it, and it has
to be *my* action, not someone else's. I realize that surgery or
chemotherapy or radiation is my action in a very real sense
because it's my decision. In the actual doing, however, it is the
action of others—researchers and pharmacists and nurses and
physicians. If I stop at only cooperating with or accepting their
actions, I haven't really made the commitment to fighting cancer.

Every day, Emmett Kelly, the sad-faced clown, comes and
sweeps all the cancer cells out of my body. Remember his little
broom? I call it the light broom. Actually, there was a circle of
light on the floor. As Kelly swept, the electrical technician made
the circle smaller and smaller, making it appear that the clown's
broom was sweeping up the light. While I'm in the bathtub, I have
Emmett go through my whole body, sweeping with his little circle
of light. (If you've read the meditation on singing on page 15,
you'll remember that visualization and music can work together

43

nicely.) By the time he's done, all the cancer cells are gone. That visualization is something I do that no one else can do for me.

We are really committed when we take the actions that are available to us alone: visualization, meditation, biofeedback, attending healing services, talking to ourselves, learning more about our disease and treatment so we have better control, body monitoring, prayer, giving ourselves the right messages for health, eating correctly, exercising, avoiding tobacco and alcohol, finding occasions for laughter each day, reducing stress, laying healing hands on our own bodies.

Not all of these are for everyone. However, the more of them that we can do for ourselves, the greater our own sense of commitment, and the better we then feel about ourselves. That in turn increases the peace and reduces the stress in our bodies, giving our healing agents room to work.

Research was done on women having breast biopsies. The group that reacted best was those whose first action and attitude were prayer. Faith, whether religious or otherwise, provides control. The faith of these women gave them control, which allowed them to make the commitment to action in prayer. That action reduced the level of stress hormones.

Another way the stress hormones are reduced is involvement with helping others—in a support group, in volunteer work, in someone's personal care. The way to health is not only commitment to doing the things that get me well but commitment to action that makes healthy the society and environment around me.

Commitment is determination and action stuck together, like peanut butter and bread. It is both seeing the goal and kicking the ball toward it.

I used to run with a young woman who liked everything about running—except running. She was great at talking about it, reading running magazines, buying running clothes and shoes, stretching out. When it came to hitting the road, though, she didn't really want to do it. She liked the idea, but she wasn't committed.

Getting well takes commitment, which isn't easy. It surely is rewarding, though!

Now that I have cancer, I'm committed.

. . . *I am whole.*

AT LEAST, I AM more whole than I've been before.

On the face (or the colon) of it, that sounds silly. *Hole* looks more accurate than *whole*. After all, a part of me is missing. Strangely, now I am more whole.

Connectedness is the key to wellness: connectedness to others, to one's own self, to purpose. In other words, wholeness—putting it all together.

The less connected we are, the less together, the less whole and well we are. All the parts of us that are not integrated into the whole have more chance of getting sick because they're out there by themselves, with no support, no surrounding buttresses of love and solidarity.

There's a story about a man who fell into the river. An old sailor rowed out to him. Just as the man was about to go under, the sailor grabbed his arm. But it was an artificial arm and came off in the sailor's hands. The man went under again, but when he came up, the sailor grabbed his hair. Unfortunately, the man wore a wig, and it, too, came off in his hands. When the man rose yet again, the old salt grabbed his clothes and shouted, "How can I save you if you won't stick together?"

We've got to stick together if we want to get well. That means we integrate mind, body, and spirit. The best mark of a long-term survivor is the integration—into wholeness—of love and attitude and looking for purpose and exercise and diet and spirituality and laughter and appreciation for life and relationships and self-love and seeing new options and learning new ways.

We don't have to have all these in place when we start. They are all approaches that can be learned. Wellness often is a matter of finding new options, seeing in ways we haven't been trained to see. Working hard at learning and integration does the immune system more good than any other therapy.

Cancer is a spiritual disease because it requires us to face the dilemma of fragmentation and wholeness. In our culture we are used to the adversarial system, whether it is lawyer versus lawyer in the justice system, cop versus criminal on the streets, cowboy versus Indian in the movies, man versus woman in marriage, team versus team on the athletic field, management versus labor in the workplace. There must be a loser for each winner. Someone has to be "number one," and that's the only number that counts.

In trying to beat cancer, however, I am competing against myself. Cancer is a part of me, so if I win, I also lose. Getting whole, getting well, has to do with oneness. It's not a matter of right or wrong, victory or defeat, not even life or death. It is life versus nonlife. If I experience wholeness in life, death is not a defeat. If I experience fragmentation in life, then life is not a victory.

The goal, the sense of purpose, is not so much getting cured, beating the cancer, continuing to live. The goal is wholeness itself, being a full and complete person. That is adequate purpose. In fact, it is the only worthy purpose of life. I don't have to make some great achievement, do some mighty work, to justify my existence. Being a whole person *is* the purpose for our being.

There is no single road to wellness. Getting well and being well is taking an interlocking network of highways that lead to the one, central junction of wholeness.

Cure is an end result concept. Wellness, health, healing, wholeness—these are process, each-moment-at-a-time concepts. I don't just want to be cured, to reach the end of one road. I want to be whole for each moment of all my life, whether my days are few or many.

Sickness, especially from cancer, often produces spirituality. One reason is because we are taught visualization, meditation, and prayer as methods for increasing our body's healing agents, enhancing our immune system. I think there's something spiritual about cancer itself, though. It's a challenge to wholeness, to the integration of love. If we take the challenge of cancer, we almost have to face our fragmentation and begin to pull together the scattered pieces of our selves.

Now that I have cancer, I am whole.

. . . *I've got an attitude.*

THEY SAY YOU HAVE a better chance if you have a good attitude. I'm not sure about that. I suspect the most important thing is just to have an attitude. Your own attitude. Period.

There is a man in my support group. His name is Jim. He's had cancer twice. They told him the first time he wouldn't live a year. The second time he lost a lung. He's convinced he'll get it a third time—if he lives that long. He's been going around with a bad attitude for five years. He's proud of it.

"They say you've got to have a good attitude. Ridiculous! I've got the worst attitude there is, and I'm still here!"

Jim really grooves on "havin' a 'tude," as the saying goes. He doesn't feel the need for any "attitude adjustment," either. He's baaaaad, and he's glaaaaad!

Jim doesn't have what anyone could describe as a good attitude, but he has a great attitude for dealing with cancer. He's so proud of living with a bad one that he keeps on going just to prove it can be done. It gives him a reason to keep fighting. He's got a cause. He's accepted the challenge. He's made the commitment. He's out to prove you don't have to have a good attitude to deal with cancer, which is a good attitude to take. He'll do it even if it means he has to live.

What we really need is a cancer attitude, not a good attitude. "Anything that works," that's the cancer motto. Cancer is a very personal disease. Each of us must deal with it in his or her own best way.

Bernie Siegel says he can always tell when a patient is going to get well. It's when a nurse or another physician has marked "Bad Attitude" on the chart. It means the patient is taking responsibility. In other words, the patient is not being "cooperative," isn't doing what makes life easier for the nurses, technicians, and physicians.

I'm very open about having cancer, and about my treatment, and about my pains, and about, well, just everything about the disease. That's difficult for some people. It scares them. They don't even want to hear the word, let alone hear about what it's like.

One man told me about his friend, Dan.

"Dan got cancer," he said, "but he never talked about it. Why, you'd never even know he had it. He just went right on with life as usual."

"He sounds like a good man," I said. "I'd like to meet him."

"Uh, well, you can't. He's dead, but you'd never know he had it, right up to the day he died."

With no blame on Dan, he's not a good model for me. I don't want to be like him. He's dead.

How many times have you heard an ill person, whether with cancer or arthritis or another debilitating disease, extolled in words like these: "Oh, she never complains. Even when she's feeling her worst, if you ask her how she is, she always smiles and replies, 'Just fine.'"

I'm not going to argue with those folks. Like I said, it's a personal disease. Each of us has to take the attitude we think is best for us. If you say "I'm just fine" when you're hurting, that's just fine, as long as it's your decision, your real attitude. But is it your decision? Is it your attitude, or is it the attitude someone else has decided you ought to take?

I admire folks who do the best they can with what they've got, even if it's not much. There's a way in which each of us ought to be able to say "Just fine," regardless of how much we're hurting. "Just fine" is a relative term. My condition might not be acceptable for you, but it's "just fine" for me.

That is for me to decide for me—and for you to decide for you. The best attitude is the one that is true and genuine, the one that really is mine, the one that really is yours—not the one that is the most convenient and nonthreatening for others.

Now that I have cancer, I've got an attitude,
and it's mine.

4. WHEN YOU'RE BALD AND STRANGELY BEAUTIFUL

(TREATMENT)

Now that I have cancer . . .

. . . *I'm my own hero.*

BERNIE SIEGEL SAYS THAT disease gives us a chance to live out our personal myths and become heroes. I have many personal myths: baseball star, jazz bassoonist, great writer. The most enduring one, though, is that I am a runner.

I've always thought of myself as a long-distance runner. I've not always been one, you understand, but I've always thought of myself that way. In grade school, I thrilled as Glenn Cunningham made his assaults on the "unbreakable" four-minute barrier for the mile run. In those days, most people considered a mile long-distance running. When I went out for track in high school, I decided to double the heroics by running the 2-mile race. Later, when I was a road runner, 10-kilometer (6.2-mile) races were popular. Gradually I worked up to the marathon: 26 miles, 385 yards.

We distance runners are, on the whole, a disdainful lot. We like to say things like, "Oh, you need me there in thirty minutes and it's ten miles? Well, my wife has the car, but I'll just run over." (Don't bother to figure up the arithmetic; it will only confuse you.) Or we put slogans on our shirts like, "When the going gets tough, the sprinters stop." We tend to think that our many miles will save us from all health problems, except sore feet, shin splints, aching joints, and sagging breasts, of course. We assume we'll never die; we'll just run off into the sunset someday and not return. We are, quite simply, arrogant in our health. We work at it, but we assume that work is a guarantee. Consequently, we're not prepared when our bodies get cancer or heart disease. "But look at all those miles I put in," we want to wail.

Now I find those miles work for me in a different way. With a chemo habit on my back and a Groshong catheter in my chest, I'm just a slow walker these days, not the distance runner I thought I was. But I *have* been there. I have seen the finish line after twenty-six miles. I know I can do a marathon because I have done a marathon.

So I divided my fifty-two weeks of chemotherapy up into fifty-two half-mile segments of a marathon. I said to myself, "I know I can complete this chemo course because I can complete any marathon course." Half mile by half mile, I have done it. I know what it is to hit the wall, in either marathon. I know what it is to ache so bad that all I want to do is quit, in either marathon. But I have run them both, and I have finished the course.

I've always thought of myself as a long-distance runner. Now that I have cancer, I think of myself as a long-distance victor. And a hero.

. . . *I'm superstitious.*

I'VE NEVER BEEN SUPERSTITIOUS before. Oh, I always wear my Hoosiers cap with the bill cocked to the left when I watch Indiana University basketball games, but that's just fun. I don't really think it affects the score. Now, however, I want so much to do the right things and avoid the wrong things—the actions and even the thoughts that might determine whether my cancer goes or stays.

When I go in for a chemo treatment, I sit in the chair where my vein puckered up best to take the IV needle. I know the chair didn't have anything to do with it, but I'm taking no chances. I had a banana for breakfast before my last chemo treatment, and I didn't get sick. I've had so many breakfast bananas since then, I'm beginning to walk like a chimp. Maybe bananas are just good sense instead of superstition. But what about the plaid shirt phenomenon? I don't get mouth sores on days I wear plaid to chemo. You think I'm going to take a chance on a plain shirt? No way!

I'm an amateur magician. I love to make children laugh and wonder how in the world I made the three ropes into one or made the ball disappear and then come out Patty's ear. Magic is fun. It's not wise to take it seriously, though. I can't put cancer into my red velvet bag and make it go away. I can't cause it to disappear up my sleeve by saying "Abracadabra."

So what's the difference between being superstitious and simply acknowledging the mysterious nature of life? Where does faith trail off into magic? What is good sense and what is just silliness? What is the right thing?

I'm not sure there is a right thing—a right chair to sit in, or shirt to wear, or even food to eat. But if there is no right thing to do, how will I get well? Is my health really just a matter of chance? Is there nothing I can do to help?

I suspect there are right things to do, but they are not in the realm of chairs or shirts or even bananas. They have more to do with faith than magic, prayer than potions, good thoughts than correct rituals. Sometimes, though, we need to express our own faith in the future, and in the present, by acting out our fears and hopes. If I wear a plaid shirt and sit in the same chair each time in the chemo room, I'm saying that I'm not just a victim. I'm not a withering leaf, blown by whatever wind has the most bluster. I have choices to make, and those choices make a difference.

I can choose love instead of fear, wholeness rather than fragmentation, relationship over loneliness, control instead of dependence. Those choices are never easy, but they are possible. One way I remind myself that I can make those choices is by which shirt I wear and which chair I sit in. My superstitions are signs of hope.

Now that I have cancer, I'm superstitious, and hopeful.

. . . *I'm waiting for "the last drop on the last day."*

THAT'S THE ONE, MY oncologist assures me, that makes the cure.

Of course, my oncologist is a bit of a comedian. "Does it hurt yet?" he asks me as he installs the Groshong catheter in my chest. "No," I tell him. "Darn," he says. "I must be doing something wrong." At least, I *think* he's a comedian.

He keeps giving me the "last drop" theory to keep me going. My side effects were so bad the first month of chemotherapy: mouth sores to the point I couldn't eat or talk; diarrhea out the . . . well, that goes without saying; eyes watering and gluing themselves shut and going out of focus; veins inflamed; hands and feet swelling so bad I couldn't walk for a couple of days.

One dark night at 2 A.M. I promised myself I could quit at the end of six months, instead of going the whole twelve, if they didn't get better. The problem is that I'm part of a clinical trial. It would mess up the statistics if I quit early. He keeps making me wait for the last drop on the last day.

I'm glad he does. I want to be part of the clinical trial. I want my pain to be useful in learning things that will be valuable in treating others.

Maxwell House used to advertise its coffee as "good to the last drop." I have no doubt that chemo will be bad to the last drop, but I'm going to keep going, and not just because I'll mess up somebody's statistics.

There's an old story from the river country close to where I grew up. The waters rose in the spring, as they always did, flooding the countryside and driving people up onto the rooftops. One whole family was up there, watching things float by—a tree, a chicken coop, a pig, an old hat. But the old hat stopped at the edge of their yard and turned around and went back upstream, against the flood. At the other edge, it stopped again, turned and came back down. Back and forth it went, with the water, then against the water, as the family sat and wondered what strange phenomenon could have caused this unlikely sight. Then one of the boys slapped his head and exclaimed, "I remember now. Grandpa said he was going to mow the yard today, come hell or high water."

There are some things that you do just because you have to. Our younger daughter, Katie, says that is the best thing I ever told her, which is pretty good considering what she usually thinks of my advice.

"You've told me a lot of lies," she says.

"What do you mean? How could I ever have told you a lie?"

"Well, for instance, you always said, 'You'll understand it better when you're older.' I'm older now, but I don't understand things any better. But when I went to college, you said, 'There are some things you have to do just because you have to do them. You don't have to feel like doing them or want to do them or have the right circumstances for doing them. You just have to do them.' That's gotten me through a lot of tough jobs."

Someone surmised to the Duke of Wellington after his defeat of Napoleon at Waterloo that the English soldiers must have been braver than the French soldiers to have won the victory.

"No," replied Wellington, "the French soldiers were brave. But the English soldiers were brave five minutes longer."

I suspect that's often the case—not how brave or smart you are but how long you use the intelligence and courage given you.

Now that I have cancer, I'm going for the last drop on the last day.

. . . I'm trying to learn to be a complainer.

COMPLAINERS GET WELL BETTER. They get all their negative feelings out, get all those emotional toxins out of their system. You ever heard of a prize fighter who got cancer? Of course not. They might be a little loopy, but they don't have any aggression or hostility turned inward on themselves. They get it all out on the heads of other people.

Some complainers do that, too, which is why we're taught not to complain. So many people make complaining into a nasty business, by dumping their dis-ease all over everyone else, instead of dropping it off at the safe emotional nuclear waste dump. So from the time we are little children, we are told we should keep a stiff upper lip, be a brave boy or girl, or a "big" one, knowing that "big" boys and girls don't cry, and not bother other people with our complaints about life.

Thank goodness Helen and I were unsuccessful with our daughters. We tried and tried to make them stoic uncomplainers. They would have nothing of it. A neighbor once named our older daughter, then about eight, "Mary Too." Mary was always too hot or too cold, too tall or too short, too hungry or too full, too rich or too poor. The world was too light or too dark. She was "Mary Too." Too much of a complainer, her parents felt, but she had built-in good instincts, for which we are very grateful. A child's good instincts make up for a lot of bad parenting.

So now I'm trying to learn from my children. I'm complaining, in safe ways and safe places. I go to cancer support group. I attend prayer circle at church. I tell God all about it. I walk it off, muttering complaints with every step. Everybody in town knows about my watery eyes. When someone asks me how I am, they find out. (If they don't want to know, they shouldn't ask.)

Even saying all that embarrasses me, though. I'm not a complaining type. I know there are so many people who have it worse than I do. What do I have to complain about? I've always gotten my points from being a "nice" person, one who caused no strain or pain to others. Down deep, I still think that's the way a person is supposed to be. But thank God for my family and friends. They say, "Hey, lean on us. You don't have to be nice all the time. We love you regardless. If you hurt, you tell us. If you don't like having cancer, good for you. Complain and get well. We'd rather have a complaining and alive you than just a 'nice' memory."

One of my chemo-pushing nurses said one day, "Now you listen. This is no competition to see who can stand the most pain. If I hurt you, you tell me." She's right, as chemo nurses always are. This isn't a niceness contest. This is a getting-well struggle, and I'm going to win, even if I have to kick a little . . . well, niceness habit.

Have I told you about my diarrhea? No? Well, just wait until you hear this. . . .

Now that I have cancer, I'm learning to be a complainer.

. . . *My morning misery has become a joy.*

IT DIDN'T START OUT that way. In fact, I didn't even have a morning misery until I had cancer.

I've always been a morning person. I love to get up with the sun and the roosters, sip a cup of tea, run five miles, have some time for myself. Unfortunately, I'm also a night person. I love to stay up late, reading good novels and watching bad TV. Being both a morning person and a night person is a bad combination; it's hard to get any sleep, especially if the people who are paying you expect you to work during the day.

Now I'm neither a morning nor a night person. I'm so tired I can't stay up late. Sometimes I sleep ten hours and feel no more rested when I get up than when I went to bed. Worst of all, though, is what happens to my insides in the morning.

They removed one-third of my colon to get that malignant tumor out, then resectioned it. That changed my bowel habits. (Noncancer folks might think this isn't polite to talk about, but it's the real world for us, right?) Ever since, I get thirty to ninety seconds' notice before I have to be seated, and I don't mean at a table. When it happens, I don't want to be very far from a bathroom.

This severely reduced bowel, what I call my semicolon, moves four or five times in the first three or four hours after I get up in the morning, with no more than a warning of a minute and a half to me. That's more movements than a symphony. It might even be more times than that if the chemo has given me diarrhea. In addition, in the aftermath of surgery, I've had trouble with hemorrhoids, something I never before experienced. After each movement, I have to get undressed, get in the shower, and "cleanse myself thoroughly and gently." Now with that combination, I'm sure you understand when I use the term "morning misery."

So why do I say it's a joy? Because I've gotten acquainted with Bernie Siegel and Joan Borysenko and Norman Cousins and Greg Anderson and Gerald May and Regina Sara Ryan and Mary McDermott Shideler in the process. There's a little table in my bathroom, one my father made. On it are piled their books. I don't allow myself to read them except when I'm in the bathroom. It makes me look forward to my period of morning misery.

These folks are my friends and soul physicians. They speak to me the wisdom I need to hear. Some of them I had heard of vaguely before. Others are brand new to me. Some of the books have been given to me or recommended to me by friends. Others I have found browsing bookstore shelves. (Not in the morning, of course.)

My life is so enriched by these new friends. I can't imagine what I would do without our daily chats. Each day I learn new coping skills. I learn how to live fully within the limits I'm now given. With their guidance I feel more deeply into my own life and the love that is there for me in the presence of others.

Beethoven said that if he had to choose between the joys and sorrows of his life, he would keep the sorrows, because he had learned so much more from them. I understand what he meant. If I had to lose my new friends to get rid of my morning misery, I would keep the misery.

I'm not just trying to avoid the morning misery by being transported into the realm of books so I can mask out what is actually happening to me. I stay in the moment, even the moment of distress. But these authors participate in the present with me. It's not avoidance of the pain and discomfort, but the misery is diminished by being shared.

Of course, I could read Bernie and Joan and Gerald and Mary and the others at some other time. However, that would not change my morning routine, and my misery would be only that: misery.

I suspect it's better to have misery one can share with friends than to have joy and no one with whom to share it. That's why, now that I have cancer, my morning misery is a joy.

... I get sick when I see Becky.

BECKY IS THE HEAD nurse in the cancer clinic. She's my pusher, inserting that needle, pushing that chemo into me. I like Becky. She's competent and pleasant and very pretty. I could look at her all day, except for one thing: She makes me sick!

You've probably heard this kind of story already, so here are some more.

Marie, a nurse practitioner at my cancer clinic, a lovely and sophisticated lady, came around the corner of an aisle in a grocery store one day. She came face to face with a clinic patient. The woman promptly threw up all over poor Marie.

An American oncologist walking down a street in Paris saw a woman coming toward him. She suddenly doubled up and started vomiting in the gutter. He hurried to her to see whether he could help. Then he recognized her, from back in the States. She was a former chemo patient. He hadn't seen her for eight years! One look at his face, though, even in a foreign country, and there went the cookies.

I have a friend who munches crackers on her forty-five-mile drive to her chemo treatments. As soon as she gets into the car and heads north out of her town, she feels the nausea coming on. The crackers help keep it down.

So we come back to the ever-gracious Becky, who's been enduring tales like this for the fifteen years of her oncology nursing practice. I park in the garage. I walk across the street, down the stairs, into the long tunnel over to the cancer clinic. With every step the nausea level rises higher.

Finally, I walk into the clinic, see Becky, and run like mad for the restroom, to call Ralph on the big white phone. (Isn't it amazing, the number of euphemisms we have for vomiting?)

It's called anticipatory nausea. It reminds us that we are a unity of body and mind. Nothing has been put into my body yet, to make me sick, when I walk in and see Becky. In fact, I'm as far away from my last nauseating treatment as I'll ever be, so I ought to be at my best, right? No way! My mind knows what's coming. It has a reason, even if my body doesn't.

Some people say that it's silly to get sick, or feel pain, when your body hasn't yet been subjected to it. "It's all in your head," they say, as though what's in your head doesn't count.

What's in your head does count, and the count goes even higher when you add what's in your nose and taste buds and ears and eyes. William Redd, a psychologist who's done a great deal of research in this area, is a consultant to fragrance manufacturers. He says, "If you want to sell your perfume, don't let a nurse wear it."

There are ways we can neutralize the anticipatory nausea and pains: hypnosis, meditation, relaxation techniques, imaging. Some hospitals and cancer clinics have even begun to teach these. Probably the most simple is just to put yourself, in your mind, some place you'd rather be.

When I park in the garage now, it's the same one I parked in across from Riverfront Stadium where I went to see the Reds play. When I walk that long tunnel, it's the gangway across the street to the blue seats. Then I step into the clinic, and there they are, watching for me in the waiting room, cheering that I have finally arrived to save the game: Joe Morgan and Chris Sabo and Johnny Bench and Pete Rose, you bet.

The mind is a great gift from God, with its ability to imagine, to be playful. If we get careless with it, it can get us into a lot of trouble, but it can also be the way of healing. Anticipatory nausea reminds us that we are whole creatures, and we need to be healed as a whole, mind and body both, together.

I'll admit that Becky looks a little strange in a Reds uniform, but at least she's not nauseating!

. . . *I am blessed.*

I LEARNED THAT FROM a young man in the cancer center. No, not a doctor, nor a nurse, nor a fellow patient. The janitor.

One nauseated and cold chemo day I left my car in the hospital parking garage and started the long walk through the underground tunnel to the cancer center. Step by step—I knew what was waiting. Step by step, closer to the verge. Yes, you know the verge I mean, "the urge to regurge," as we said as children. And not a toilet or sink in sight.

Self-pity swirled around me like a pernicious fog, the thick kind of fog the Scots call the dreaded *haar*. Dread like a stone in the belly.

I was just about to decorate the wall with my breakfast when the janitor appeared from around the bend in the tunnel, pulling a big cart full of rubbish. Well, you really hate to throw up in the hallway when the one who has to clean it up is standing right there, so I took a deep breath and started to go on.

"How are you today?" he asked, eyes flashing and teeth gleaming.

It was clearly a good day for him. I resented his obvious vitality and robust health. He looked like he could eat a pickled Chevrolet and never burp. So I decided to answer his question truthfully.

We do that sometimes, don't we? We tell the truth as revenge. As my nun friend, Sister Thecla, says, "Sing loudly. That way we can get back at God for giving us these voices."

People say, "How are you?" and expect to hear an automatic "Fine." Well, I wasn't fine, and I told him so.

"I'm miserable," I mumbled.

He sobered up immediately, his ear cocked toward me like a collie. Then I felt a little guilty. After all, he was just being pleasant. It wasn't fair to put him on the spot like that.

So I did the usual. I asked him back, "How are you?"

With a remarkable combination of dignity and joy and compassion, he replied, "Blessed!"

"Blessed!" What a happy expression.

You know, it didn't do a thing for my nausea. I went on down the hall and threw up in the bathroom. I assume the blessed janitor had to clean it up.

Blessings are not just a matter of how we feel at the moment, although I'll be the first to admit that a day without pain and fatigue and side effects is a blessing all by itself. The blessings are there for the taking, even if the miseries have caught us by the hair and started yanking. As I hugged the porcelain deity, I said, "Yeah, I'm blessed, even now, because God loves me, and I have people who love me. He's right. I'm blessed, too."

Blessed. Blessed with the efforts of researchers and physicians and laboratory workers and nurses. Blessed by people who never knew me but who taught my physicians and passed on to my nurses their caring values. Blessed with the love of people who pray for me and care for me. Whatever recovery I may have is a gift from generations of loving people. I'm blessed.

I was blessed by the truth, too. I told him how I really felt instead of giving some glib "Okay," and it was therapeutic. Yes, sometimes we tell the truth for revenge, but saying "I'm fine" when we're not doesn't help us get well. It's the truth that makes us free to receive the blessings.

I am blessed by a young janitor, whose simple witness reminds me that life is a gift, even when I'm about to get wrung inside out by the chemo bends.

Now that I have cancer, I am blessed.

. . . *I'm sick and tired of being sick and tired.*

BEING TIRED DEPRESSES ME. Even the simplest tasks are hard to do. The tiredness and depression are mostly from the chemo, I know, but I have almost a year of that to go. Just about the time I get a little energy back, I have to go back for more chemo. I'm just so sick and tired of being sick and tired.

Nothing works right, either. My eyes, eyes that used to pick out a fly ball at a hundred yards, are so bad. The lids are stuck together most of the time. My friend Jack Newsome was up on the leadership platform at a meeting we both attended. I was in the front row. We've been the best of friends for years, and we weren't more than twenty feet apart, but I could barely make him out, barely pick him out from the others sitting up there.

It's not just my eyes. My hands and feet are swollen. My mouth is sore. I can't shave or use tools or go to the dentist for fear of meeting a germ or getting a cut. I spend half the day in the bathroom. If I get a whiff of the wrong smell, I'll toss my cookies. The problem is that the odors take turns being the wrong one. I never know which smell is the wrong one until it's too late. For two weeks after chemo I can only eat white stuff: potato soup and tapioca and crackers and pasta without sauce. I long for colored food!

I'm sick and tired of thinking about cancer, too. I'm sick of hearing about it and reading about it.

I have stacks of color-coded paper with instructions on how to deal with the side effects of my chemotherapy. Nurses and doctors and strangers on the street give me advice and information and orders. Books and pamphlets pile up beside my place at the table, and more arrive daily in the mail.

I don't want to be a cancer expert. I just want to be done with it. I want to read Anne Tyler, not Bernie Siegel. I want to go to ball games, not support groups. Nurses are wonderful, but I never want to see a white dress again. I want to hear a mechanic say, "Your transmission's shot," rather than hear a nurse say, "This vein's shot." I want to be a good old boy and drive my pickup and drink real coffee down at the oasis and talk about the price of soybeans. I want to be "normal."

I wasn't prepared for all this. I went to get a second opinion from an oncologist who was recommended to me by a friend. For a long time they called him "Dr. Cancer" because he was the best at beating that word down. Then they got used to him, so now they just call him Dr. Hatfield.

He said, "You need to be in this clinical trial, a year's worth of new chemo drugs for your type of cancer. The problem is that you have to start it within thirty days of your surgery, and this is your thirtieth day. So, take your time, and think about it, but I have to leave for a board meeting in fifteen minutes."

I just didn't get much time to get ready. I'd had no symptoms when I had the surgery. Then I had fifteen minutes to decide on chemo. I've been around cancer patients a lot in my life, but they weren't in my family, and certainly I've never been one before. I just wasn't prepared for how tired I am, how sore this is making me.

Cancer cells are fast-dividing cells. Basically the chemotherapy drugs have to attack all the fast-dividing cells, killing them all, on the theory that the healthy ones, the noncancerous ones, will regenerate. I didn't know I had so many speedy little cells: stomach and intestines and mouth and hair and palms and soles, and especially the energy cells. Those guys have really been knocked for a loop.

I think back, though, to looking for Jack, up on the platform, through my chemo-fuzzed eyes, and this is what I remember: For all the fuzziness, he still looked like my friend. It's difficult ever to have clear vision, with or without chemo. If you can recognize your friends, though, you're okay.

All those mouth sores and eye sores and foot sores—they're ways of recognizing my friends. They let me know that the chemo is doing its job, separating out the cells we don't want, letting the others have a chance to take up the room they need without being crowded out.

Now that I have cancer, I'm sick and tired of being sick and tired, but I know that, one way or another, there's a new day comin'. I'm just thankful for my friends, all of them.

. . . *I'm a prisoner in my own house.*

NOT ENTIRELY, OF COURSE. There are times when I must leave, most notably on the five-days-in-a-row intravenous chemotherapy weeks. There are other days when I can get out, even days when I can go to work.

But I can't be in the sunshine; the chemo's made my skin too sensitive for that. I can't go to church or to the mall or the theater if infections are lurking in the air; the chemo's suppressed my immune system too much for that. I can't hold a baby unless I've first been assured it hasn't had any recent vaccinations.

So I'm a prisoner in my own house. That bothers me. I don't want to think of my house as a prison. I like my house. It's always been a refuge, like a game preserve for an endangered species, which, perhaps, I am.

My house has big windows and lots of light. Flowering crab trees bloom just outside the glass. Squirrels and birds come right up to the ends of the branches and look in. Plants bloom around the living room. Pictures of family give me my history as I walk down the hall. Hundreds of books live here, piled on the tops of tables my father has crafted even though he's blind. Music boxes sing one to another from room to room. Puzzles and games and little horse statues remind us of when our girls still lived here. There's a grim and terrible contradiction in being a prisoner in paradise.

Sometimes now my house seems like a colonial blockhouse or western fort. I'm hunched down in here below the firing slits, trying to escape the savages that besiege our walls with their catapults and arrows and cannon. The problem is, the savages are in here, too. In fact, they are already inside of me. We're prisons within prisons. I'm a prisoner in my house, and the cancer

71

cells are prisoners within the house of my body, trying so hard to escape that they are running rampant.

I wonder what they're so afraid of, why they started forting up in tumors, imprisoning themselves within me. Do they see the contradiction, too, of being a prisoner in a place that's meant for love and hope and beauty instead of for fear and being shut in? Prisoners and their guards always have to live together, just as the cancer cells and I do.

We are all prisoners in some way, to something. The trick of life surely is to choose your prison well. My cancer cells and I have both chosen wisely in many ways. I cannot think of a better place to be a prisoner than in my house. Apparently they could not think of a better place for imprisonment than in the house of my body.

Houses and bodies are not meant to be jails, however. I want to be released from my house so that it can be a home again instead of a stockade. I want my cancer cells to be freed, too. I want them to be released from the fearful compulsion that makes them multiply so quickly so that they, also, can become normal, free, hopeful cells again and live within me as within a home rather than as bolted down and penned in, afraid of what lies outside.

Now that I have cancer, I'm a prisoner in my own house, but I have company, and we are all working to be free.

5. WHEN THE NIGHT FRIGHTS COME

(THINKING ABOUT DEATH)

Now that I have cancer . . .

. . . I have to walk that lonesome valley by myself.

THAT'S WHAT THE OLD spiritual says: "Jesus walked that lonesome valley, had to walk it by himself. Oh, nobody else could walk it for him, had to walk it by himself." Then it reminds us that each of us has to walk that lonesome valley alone as well, "have to walk it by yourself."

When I first heard that word, *cancer*, and I thought I would be dead from it very soon, the idea of walking that lonesome valley all by myself simply terrified me. I'd never thought about it before. Oh, I've certainly thought about death. You can't even see a Woody Allen movie without thinking about death. We all know that no one gets out of this life alive. But I had never realized how lonesome it would be.

I had a hospital roommate, a very nice man. Nurses and other hospital personnel streamed in and out of the room like worker ants. Friends dropped by every day, so many that my wife installed a turnstile in the doorway and made them show passes. Helen and Mary Beth and Katie must have put in twenty-four hospital hours per day between them. Still, I was in a darkening valley of pain and fear all by myself. None of those other folks, the ones in regular clothes who could eat regular food, none of them was on death's waiting list. I was the one, and it scared the hell out of me. In many ways, it still does.

That fear tells me something very important about myself. Too much of the meaning for my life comes from outside of me. I live for others—for their approval and friendship and affirmation. I've spent most of my life walking paths that will cause others to like me, or at least respect me. But that lonesome valley, that's one trip I've got to make all by myself. No amount of approval from others makes any difference. To negotiate that lonesome valley successfully, you've got to have your internal compass working, the one that points you straight at yourself, because no one else will be there.

The results of looking away from ourselves for meaning are addictions. Addictions are always based on the mistaken idea that we can get meaning for life from something other than our own selves, be it drugs or booze or money or sex or power or nicotine or thought patterns or exercise or rituals or food—you name it. We don't sit down one day and say, "I don't think I can get meaning from myself, so I'll form an addiction to something," but that's still the reason those habits get their hold on us.

Bernie Siegel says that our pain is a reset button. If we never feel the pain, we never push the button to get our lives reset. And what is it we say about addictions? "He was feelin' no pain." The addiction masks our fear and uncertainty, even if it's a "positive" addiction, such as reading or running or helping people or being nice. We've got to feel the pain, or we don't know how we've given up all the internal meaning, how we're looking to the rest of the world to make life worthwhile for us.

I think that's why Jesus was successful as a healer in some cases and not in others. Some folks were ready to have their reset buttons pushed and some were not.

Cancer has pushed my reset button. I can't live for others anymore. I don't mean I want to become selfish. There's a great difference between being self-centered and being centered in one's self. I have to be satisfied with me and my life, whether or not anyone else is.

Day by day now, I feel a little more comfortable with walking the lonesome valley by myself. I think that's a good sign. It means I'm beginning to understand that my justification for living is just that I'm here. My meaning comes from inside. All that I need for facing life, yes, and for facing death, God has already put into my life.

Now that I have cancer, I have to walk that lonesome valley by myself.

. . . I grieve already for the loss my death will bring to the world.

THAT CERTAINLY SOUNDS LIKE I'm entertaining a grandiose estimate of my value to the world. Not so. I'm well aware that only a precious handful will mourn my passing for very long. It is only presidents and generals, heroes and villains, composers and artists, who are remembered more than a generation, and not many of them. When my children and my tombstone have been erased by time and wind, I shall be no more to this world, not even in memory, along with billions of other bodies who have left no more mark on the earth than a leaf leaves on the storm. That must be the plan of the Creator, for it is certainly the way of all flesh.

Cancer makes us think about death, doesn't it? Even if we have every confidence that we shall recover, be cured, be saved from this particular hit man sent by the cancer Mafia, we are reminded that someday we shall die. For many of us, cancer will be the cause of death. Most of us still, the first time we hear that word applied to us, immediately think of death.

I have the normal fears of death and dying, but they are not the reason for this leap forward to grief that I am experiencing now. You see, I, and I alone, in this particular brain and body, have certain memories, specific hopes, particular clusters of relationships, my own peculiar way of seeing the world. When I am gone, the whole universe of my experience is gone. Not only are my language and my knowledge and my relationships gone, but all the effort I put into learning to read and understand and be a friend is also no more. Who else knows how it feels to be twenty years old and hear Helen say for the first time, "I love you"? Who else remembers what it was like to be the first McFarland or Pond to receive a college diploma? Who else ever dreamed that he hit a home run to win the World Series the same day his twelve-volume *History of the World* was published?

God must be crazy to be so profligate, developing each human being, body and soul, so uniquely and completely, and then letting all that go in death. How stupid. How inefficient. Think of all that waste, all the starting over, all that's lost each time this happens. Why, you'd think the world is infinite, that space goes on forever, that God has all the time in the world, acting that way!

Is God simply experimenting with us, trying one after another until one of us finally gets it right? If one of us does finally get it right, will everyone from then on be exactly like that one? Will she or he be the pattern for all to come?

I suspect not. I think God has something else in mind. (You may not want to use the word *God* here, and that is perfectly okay, of course; substitute your own word, because it's the one you've been given in your uniqueness to use.) I am convinced, by faith but also by reason, that God is telling us something by acting in this crazy way. I think we're being told that love is at the heart of everything—space and time and life—and that love is boundless, infinite, without measure. It does not need to be conserved or reused. There is enough to go around, enough that each individual can have his or her uniqueness.

Workers in the field of addictions tell us that at the heart of any addiction is the belief that love is limited, that there isn't enough to go around, that it has to be hoarded. When one feels left out from limited love is when addictions develop, to try to fill the empty spaces.

Death, strangely, is God's way of saying it isn't so, of letting us know that love has no limits, that there is so much love to go around that each of us can have a unique life in this world and pass on without a trace of us remaining, and the level of love isn't lowered even a little bit.

Now that I have cancer, I grieve already for the loss my death will bring to the world, for I am unique; no one can replace me. But that uniqueness is also a word of love. There is great sadness in the thought of my uniqueness passing from the scene, but there is great hope in the limitlessness of love.

. . . *I get termination notices.*

I COULDN'T BELIEVE IT! I ordered a trial subscription to a cancer journal for patients. When it ran out, they sent me a termination notice! Big black letters. Black edges around the envelope.

I wrote them. "Don't you know what a 'termination notice' means to a cancer patient?" I asked. "Your whole magazine is for patients; how could you be so insensitive?" I never heard back from them. I suppose they figured it wasn't worth it; I'd probably be terminated soon, anyway.

I don't want to get a termination notice. I want to live, forever. I want everything to go on just the way it is (except for the nausea).

If I get terminated, I'll never get to be an old man, and I was so looking forward to being an old man. Not just any old man. I want to be an irascible old curmudgeon. (My wife, of course, says that I don't have to worry; I've already made it.)

You can get away with so much when you're old that you can't when you're younger. You can get discounts, too.

I've looked like an old man for a long time. I went bald and gray early. My unruly white beard makes me resemble Santa enough that strange little children ask me for toys. I've looked like I was seventy-five since I was forty-five. There's an advantage to that. If I ever do get old, people will say, "You know, he hasn't aged a bit." Then they'll think I look good for my age.

When I was forty-seven, I ran into a supermarket one day to get a can of dog food for Waggs, even though she favors people food. It was a big mistake. I had forgotten it was senior citizen day. I was trying to rush to the dog food aisle and out again, but there was a comparison convention taking place in the store.

"I can remember when this dog food can was only forty-nine cents," someone would say.

A voice would come from over in the hot cereal section. "That's nothing; I remember when it was only thirty-nine cents."

It was like an auction. "Thirty-four. Twenty-nine. Twenty-five. Twenty-two? Anyone for twenty-two? Twenty-five once. . . . "

I grabbed a can of Cycle Old Dog and ran to the checkout lane. A young woman who couldn't have been more than a year out of high school was running the items through the scanner.

"That'll be fifty-six, with the discount."

"What discount?" I asked, assuming there must be a good looks discount or great body discount.

"Why, it's senior citizens' day," she replied. "You get the senior citizens' discount, don't you?"

I wanted to shout, "How old do you think I am?" I decided against it, though. I was afraid she might tell me.

You know what I do now? If they give me the discount without asking whether I'm eligible, I take it. I figure it's compensation for pain and suffering. I also figure it's one way I can get to be an irascible old curmudgeon, regardless of how long I live.

I guess I objected to getting the discount because it was a little termination notice, a way of saying someone thinks I'm a day closer to death. But you know, they're right. I am.

Each of us is, regardless of the state of our health. Every day is a termination notice.

That makes me rethink this whole notion. If each day is a termination notice, then I do want to keep on getting them.

I've spent my life making memories for other people. When I'm finally terminated, I want folks to fill the gap of my presence with those memories. In the meantime, I'll just keep on making memories.

Now that I have cancer, I'm glad for every day and every notice.

6. WHEN YOU'RE

THE DOCTOR

(TAKING RESPONSIBILITY)

Now that I have cancer . . .

. . . I'm the doctor.

MY SURGEON FORGOT I was in the hospital! (You can read the full story of this in the meditation on remembering where you are, on page 23.) Flat out thought I'd gone home, so he didn't come in for three days, until I had the nurse call him up to find out where he was. I'm not sure why he thought I was gone, since he hadn't dismissed me. Just busy, I guess.

I was busy, too, however—busy getting my five tubes unhooked every morning at 5 A.M. so I could stagger onto the scale to be reminded I couldn't eat, busy drinking that grape juice they strain through nuclear waste to give it that tangy taste, and then busy throwing up in that little curved pan, busy lying around waiting for the doctor to come in to take care of me.

Then an oncologist I'd never met and didn't know from a flea-bottomist came in, right after I was weighed, and told me I had "it." *"It?"* "Cancer, of course. I'll call the National Cancer Institute to see whether there's any adjuvant therapy, but I doubt it." *"Adjuvant? What does that mean?"* "You've got a 70 percent chance of recurrence in one to two years." *"Cancer? Adjuvant? What are you going to do about it?"* But he was already gone.

The surgeon forgot about me. The oncologist said there wasn't anything to do about it and that I'd be dead in a year or two.

I went to a different oncologist at another hospital. He was recommended by a friend.

"Yes," he said, "there is a therapy for you, twelve months of chemotherapy that will make you sick as a dog." (He likes to talk that medical jargon: You are either sick as a dog or healthy as a horse.) "If you're going to do it, though, we have to start today. Go out in the waiting room and talk it over with your wife."

So I sat there, bent over from the surgery, holding hands with Helen in the waiting room, a room full of thirty sick and sympathetic-looking patients, knowing I had one choice to make, that I had to make it now. She squeezed my hand and said, "For what it's worth, I know what I would do if it were my body."

If it were my body? But it wasn't *my* body! I just live in it. It's the doctors' job to take care of my body, to make it well, isn't it? But my doctor forgot me, and said there wasn't any therapy for me, and told me to take my time but do it now.

It *is* my body! It's *my* job to take care of it! *I'm* the doctor!

My surgeon is an excellent knife-wielder. My second oncologist is an excellent researcher and diagnostician and chemo-pusher. But I'm the doctor, the only one finally who has the responsibility for my body, for my life.

One thing the medical researchers have learned is that a patient deteriorates rapidly at the moment of diagnosis, the moment you get that news, that you first hear that word. It is important for the physician to tell the patient what the diagnosis is in a way that challenges but that does not hurt the possibility of recovery.

For at least two weeks after I was told I had cancer, told early in the morning by a stranger with none of my loved ones present, told that my best chance was 30 percent, I simply prepared to die. Then a lot of people who love me began to tell me, without ever saying it in so many words, "You make the diagnosis. You don't have to live with what anyone else has said, and you don't have to die with it. You're responsible for your own life. We trust you to be the doctor."

I was always the type who said to the man or woman in the white coat, with the stethoscope around the neck, "You're the doctor." We say that, don't we? If the mechanic tells us we need a new water pump, we reply, "You're the doctor." If a plumber says we need a new faucet, we say, "You're the doctor." That very phrase is part of our culture. It says that we are going to turn it over to the expert, to the "doctor" for that particular field.

Well, when it comes to me, I'm the doctor, I'm the expert, I'm the one who has to make the decisions. I need the oncologists and the radiologists and the nurses and the pharmacists, but they are *my* assistants, not the other way around. Perhaps the best thing my physician could have done for me was to forget I was in the hospital.

Now that I have cancer, I'm the doctor!

. . . *I create my own life.*

I'M THE ONLY ONE who has control of how I interpret events. I can see any occasion of my life as a bummer or as an opportunity. It will be however I see it because there is no outside, objective standard by which to judge.

For instance, no one or nothing else can make me angry. Someone else might do something I don't like or that I think is unfair, but I'm the one who decides whether I'll be angry. Your boss might fire you, your husband might leave you, your child might disappoint you, but you are the one who creates your life, not the boss or husband or child.

That's always been true, of course, but I didn't really understand it before.

Psychiatrist Viktor Frankl was a prisoner in a Nazi death camp during World War II. His wife was killed there. From that experience, he says he learned that there is one freedom no one can ever take away from you, the freedom to decide how you will react to the circumstances around you. Cancer is my death camp experience.

That makes me rethink the story of Job. Job was a good man, a blameless man. Every imaginable evil happened to Job, just so God could prove Job's faithfulness to the devil. His friends kept saying, "There must have been something you did to bring this on yourself." Job consistently protested his innocence, and he asked God for an explanation. "How come me? What did I do?" He didn't get an answer. All God said was, in effect, "If I told you, you wouldn't understand, and I'm not going to tell you, anyhow." Job never got an explanation. He could have "cursed God and died," as his friends advised, and surely he would have been justified in doing so. But he was faithful. In the face of his loss of wealth and family, in the face of his friends' sarcasm, in the face of God's arrogant silence, Job made his own decision about how he would react. He created his own life.

How I react to cancer makes all the difference. It's what I believe, what I imagine, the attitude I take, that decides whether I shall live or die. That may be true even in a physical sense, because it's often been proved that a tree's fruit is consistent. A healthy attitude makes for a healthy body. I'm speaking not just of the body, however, as important as it is, but of the spirit, where the real decisions are made, where the real life is created.

Cancer has made me see things in my life that need to be corrected. My defensiveness, for instance. In any situation—a conversation or meeting or transaction at a store—my first reaction is defensive. I expect to be criticized. I spend long hours anticipating every complaint anyone could make and then think up every possible rebuttal. This is called awfulizing, imagining the most awful situation conceivable. Of course, such detraction hardly ever happens, and if someone does find fault, it's usually not a charge I had considered anyway. Consequently, very few people have any idea how negative and self-protective I am.

I've been defensive as long as I can remember, but I had gotten used to it. I just accepted it as a part of life. Suddenly I had to ask myself, "If I have only a year or two to live, do I want to spend it being defensive?" The answer is, "No, because it's not worth it and because it won't help me get well." I'm taking charge. I'm deciding how I'll spend my mind. I'm creating my own life.

One of the marks of a long-term survivor is following a personal health plan that you think will have good results. I know there's no simple route to being well, no easy program to follow. Getting well, getting whole, comes from a whole series of small decisions. Together, though, they make up the one big decision, the choice to create your own life. When you've made that choice, you're already healed, even if your body doesn't know it.

Now that I have cancer, I create my own life.

. . . *I wonder why I got it.*

DO I HAVE SOME secret death wish? Is that why, even now, I try
to ignore it, try to go back to my old, fragmented ways of living?
They say cancer often develops in response to a loss, especially in
the previous year or two. But I can't think of any great loss that's
come my way. A little loss of energy, maybe. Some loss of ambi-
tion. My hair's been misplaced for a long time. Besides, I don't
think those are the kinds of losses the books are talking about.
They mean the loss of a loved one, or a job, or a reason to live.

I've lived a wholesome lifestyle for years: eaten a healthy
diet, loved and been loved, done meaningful work, gotten
plenty of exercise. So why did this cancer choose this year to
make its invasion?

Of course, I could claim that this cancer doesn't have anything
to do with my past lifestyle at all. It's just happenstance, or fate.

A few years ago, my eighteen- and nineteen-year-old nephews
were killed together in an auto crash, along with two of their
friends. The night of the visitation at the funeral home, the only
remaining brother of one of the other dead boys took the family
car out and managed to drive recklessly enough that he turned it
over and broke his leg.

"How could you do that?" I asked him. "Your brother is lying
dead in the funeral home. You are your parents' only living child.
Don't you have any concern, at least, for them?"

He shrugged his shoulders. "I've got no control over it," he
said. "When it's my time to go, I'll have to go."

No control over it, he said. The speed, the quick cornering,
not wearing a seat belt, not stopping at red lights—those didn't
have anything to do with whether he lived or died!

There's something appealing about that, isn't there? Life is just out of my control. I'm only the helpless subject of outside forces, whether they're the cigarettes that force themselves into my mouth or pesticides on the apricots I buy or the chemicals the Jungle Growth Company spreads on my neighbor's lawn. I have nothing to do with it, so I can't be blamed.

We live in a no-fault time, don't we? No-fault divorce, no-fault car insurance, no-fault everything. We have such a hard time handling guilt that we just legislate it out of existence until it comes in the back door under an assumed name. I want no-fault cancer.

The problem with that is that if I can't find what I did to contribute to my cancer, then I can't reverse that process to contribute to my cure. If I've got no fault, I've got no solution.

Sure, I can say outside forces caused it, so I can use outside forces such as chemotherapy and radiation to cure it. I just happen to be the man in the middle.

There's a way in which that is true. I have no doubt that outside forces helped bring about my cancer. I'm extremely grateful for the outside force of my chemotherapy. However, I can't just leave it at that.

I have to examine, at least, what I contributed, with the way I eat or the way I think, so I can change the way I eat and the way I think. I don't want to leave anything to chance. I want to have a part in getting well. I'm not just a battleground for warring armies. I'm one of the generals.

So why did I get it, especially now? I'm not sure yet,
but I thank God for the chance to wonder about it
and to work at it.

. . . I have to pay.

PAY THE PRICE FOR my own life.

The mother of a friend died. He thought his father should move into a nursing home, but the father refused. He insisted on staying in his own home. Each weekend, my friend went to his father's town, took him shopping, did the laundry, got his medicines.

After ten years, close to his death, the father said, "See, you didn't think it would work out for me to stay alone, but I've done just fine."

Shaking his head, my friend said, "He thought he had done just fine, but I was the one who didn't have a weekend for ten years. I paid the price for his lifestyle."

Who pays the price for you?

There's a great irony about price paying. The more each of us pays the price for his or her own life, the closer we are drawn together. The more each of us walks alone, the closer we walk shoulder-to-shoulder in the travels and travails of life.

Right now I'm more at one with others than I have ever been, but I'm also more alone than I've ever been.

I felt that especially in the hospital. My wife, my children, my friends, the nurses—they all did everything they could for me, but they couldn't move my bowels. They couldn't stand up and urinate for me. They could walk with me down the hall, but they couldn't take my particular, puny steps. They couldn't drink that awful, chemical-tasting grape juice for me, and I'm glad they didn't have to. It was a strange, lonesome journey, and I had to walk it by myself.

You are not real until you pay the price for your own life. Walking that lonely valley is how you pay that price. You have to take responsibility for yourself, for your own health and wholeness, even though you cannot always effect a cure for your illness any more than the doctors and nurses can.

Well, let me not talk for you. I can't say, "*You* must take responsibility." I can only say, "*I* must take responsibility for my own life." I must make the footprints of my particular journey. I can't walk yours. You can't walk mine.

There's another feeling, however, along with the aloneness: the oneness.

How is it that we are so much in oneness when each of us walks finally alone? Somehow we are never more united than when each of us is paying the price for his or her own life. I don't quite understand this, but I know it to be true.

Who pays the price for your life, for your lifestyle? We so often say to husband or wife or children or parents or friends or neighbors, "You pay. You pay for me. I can't pay. I have nothing with which to pay. You pay the price for me." We have a thousand ways to make them pay. However, when each of us says, "I'll pay my own way; I'll take the responsibility for me," then we have turned one another loose for love.

We walk alone, but as we do, we walk together. Alone, together, we walk in the courage of freedom and love.

Now that I have cancer, I have to pay the price for my own life.

7. WHEN IT'S TIME TO GIVE THANKS

(COUNTING BLESSINGS)

Now that I have cancer . . .

. . . *I never have a bad day.*

I HAVE NAUSEATED DAYS and frightened days. Tired days and hurting days. Long days and short days. Silent days and alone days. Sore mouth days and swollen hand days. Bald days and diarrhea days. Rainy days and sunny days. Cold days and warm days. But no bad days.

Every day with cancer is like a month without it. Cancer has a way of getting your attention. I sometimes say that I lived more in the first month after I found out I had cancer than I did in the previous fifty-three years. It's not that the previous fifty-three were bad years. Some elephant-sized things happened for me in those years. I got married. I fathered and helped raise my children. I made lifelong friends. I worked for good causes. However, those years went by in a blur.

My father-in-law, Earl "Tank" Karr, used to say that after age forty, the days went by at propeller speed. Suddenly you were old, and you didn't know what had become of the years.

Every cancer moment is intense. It makes you focus.

Sometimes it's the focus that the eyes of a rabbit fix on a fox, the focus of fear, the bunching of the muscles to run.

Sometimes, though, it's a focus of longing, of feeling the beauty of life so clearly that you can express it only in words of hyperbole: "Behold, you are beautiful, my love! Your eyes are doves behind your veil. Your hair is like a flock of goats, moving down the slopes of Gilead. . . . Your cheeks are like halves of a pomegranate" (Song of Solomon, chapter 4). Any woman (or man) today would think you'd slipped a gear if you tried that for romance. However, Solomon knew that even though some feelings are so strong they can't be put into words, you have to try anyway. You have to make it clear that the words you use express the depth of your emotion even though they don't make sense. Indeed, if they made sense they would only bob up on the surface, not go down deep.

Cancer brings up that sort of emotion about life and thus that inability to say in so many words what life means. When I say "I don't have a bad day," anyone outside of cancer doesn't understand. They look at me, with my puffy lips and my runny eyes and my behind so sore I can't sit down, and they say, without words, "It looks bad enough to me."

Of course it's a bad day, but it's *my* day. Every moment is full. There is no time that is idle. Each moment may be filled with fear or nausea or pain, but it is full! That's why it's not a bad moment or a bad day.

There's a story about a man who offered a $10,000 reward for the return of his wife's pet cat. His friends were astounded, for they knew that he loathed and despised that cat.

"Why are you offering so much for that cat's return when you hate it so much?" they asked.

"Ah," he said with a wink, "when you know what you know, you can afford to be extravagant."

For he knew that he had already drowned and buried his wife's pet cat!

When you know what you know, you can afford to be extravagant with each moment, living it to the fullest, putting everything you have into that one point in time, because that's all there is. I know what I know: that it is cancer that is weak and I who am strong. There's no need to hold back, to save anything for what will come, because all that might come is already here. This is the day that is, my day.

Now that I have cancer, I never have a bad day.

. . . I rejoice in my miseries.

I DON'T MEAN IN spite of my miseries; I mean *in* my miseries.

It is because of my miseries that I have been contacted by so many old friends and met so many new ones. It is because of my miseries that I have learned so much about myself and about what is important in life. It is because of my miseries that I feel I have lived more in a few months of cancer time than I did in fifty years of ordinary time. It is because of my miseries that I feel connected to love in ways I never dreamed of before.

I'm thankful for pain and side effects and disruptions in my careful schedules and new limits that hedge me in. They all sing to me a song of life. They are reminders of how precious life is.

I wrote a poem about this experience, this strange and paradoxical feeling of being thankful in misery.

> "Pain"
> And finally, now, unwanted friend,
> we die together, not alone . . .
> as we have lived.
> You are the only one who walks
> the final step with me,
> the step they claim we take,
> at last, alone.
> Until I go, you stay.
> When I go, you must.
> As long as you are with me,
> I remain.
> So no brash miracles for me,
> to snatch you far away.
> Without you, I am gone.
> As you grow stronger, I grow weak.

(Funny, that we call the weakness
growth.)
Only together do we knit the whole.
Stay awhile, if you will,
for I shall miss you. Even you, I shall miss.

I'm not romantic about pain. Sometimes it is so bad, so overpowering. It engulfs you and makes anything else, especially rejoicing, impossible. But even pain can't remain forever. And yes, I'll miss even it, because it is a reminder that I am yet alive.

There's a story about a young man who returned home after several years in military service. He was inquiring about what had happened to various people in the old neighborhood while he was away.

"Is old man Brown alive yet?" he asked.

"No, not yet," came the reply.

Life isn't automatic just because our bodies are functioning and unbroken. We don't live from birth to death but from tomb to tomb, first the tomb of the womb and then the tomb that marks the end of our particular time span on this earth. Beyond each of those tombs is the possibility of life or death.

You're not alive until you can feel the pain. Is old McFarland alive yet? Now that I have cancer, I am.

Now that I have cancer, I rejoice in my miseries.

. . . *I wear my glasses.*

THEY'RE REALLY "PLASTICS," AND I always wear them, of course. At least I do if I want to read. I can see everything else just fine without them. But not words. I bring the book up close, right against my nose, which my younger daughter has always assured me looks remarkably like a strawberry. Just a blur—the words, not my nose. I rattle and shake the newspaper until it is halfway across the room, or at least as far as my thirty-four-inch sleeve will push it. No luck—black and white but not "read all over."

Then I slip my remarkably stylish smoke gray bifocals up onto my strawberry and over my ears and "Voilà!" and "Eureka!" and all those other words that mean "Hallelujah!" I can see! Words! Not just a smudge of ink, but words.

Talk about your miracles. I slip in front of my misty blues a thin film of plastic, and immediately I'm in touch with the world: Moses and Jesus and Rousseau and old Bill Shakespeare and Tom Jefferson and Edna Ferber and Dave Barry.

Cancer's like that, isn't it? It's a lens slipped down in front of our eyes. Suddenly there's a whole new world to see. It's a strange new world, frightening in its strangeness, but there's a certain clarity, a point of focus, in all that newness.

In *The Martian Chronicles,* Ray Bradbury has a scene set in Independence, Missouri, the jumping-off point for the old wagon trains heading west. In his book, way into the future, it is the jumping-off point for people who are going off to live in space. A young woman has gone there to catch the next spaceship to Mars, to join her fiancé there. She will live the rest of her life with him on an alien planet, a place she has never seen.

She is terrified. She doesn't know whether she can go through with it. She calls him on the space telephone and pours out all her fears and doubts. He replies, but most of what he says is blanked out by static. The space telephone is not perfected, so they cannot talk back and forth. It is just her speech and then his speech, and the conversation is over.

She doesn't really know what he said. From within the garble and static, she is able to pick out only one word. In his voice, she hears the word *love*. On the strength of that one word, the next day she launches herself into space and a new life.

In all the garble of words like *levamisole* and *5-FU* and *metastasize* and *PNI* there is still a word of focus. It's always been there, but maybe we weren't wearing the right glasses to be able to see it. Cancer is a great gift if it provides the lens of love.

It's a whole new world, as scary as the thought of living on Mars, but as we see the word of love, we can take the step and go.

Now that I have cancer, I wear my glasses.

. . . *I'm thankful for the cancer.*

THE IDEA SORT OF seeped into me. No thunderclaps or lightning bolts, just a quiet awareness. I was walking, slowly, a half block farther than I'd been doing since the surgery. Enough of the nippy April morning remained that the sun's spring violet light still slanted and winked at me through first bud branches. I began to hurt, to step even slower, to worry about whether I could get home, to wonder whether I knew someone along the way who would give me a ride. It wasn't much of a context for giving thanks.

That's how it came, though, and when. I began to talk to myself, to urge myself on. Then I began to pray, to talk to God, to ask for help, for strength, just enough power and courage to push me three blocks home. I heard me say it—overheard, actually, as though it were a different person speaking: "I'm thankful for the cancer."

I guess it *was* a different person who said it.

What happens in life is that we get used to the unlovely parts. It's like having season tickets in the corner of the stadium for the football games. There's one section of the field you never see, but you get used to it, so used to your partial view that you don't even ask for better seats next year.

Or consider the floaters in front of our eyes. They obscure our vision, but most of the time we're not even aware of them. They're always there. In fact, we don't want to notice them too much, for when we do, they bother us all the more.

We go through life working and playing but not really paying attention. Cancer gets your attention. The threat of death is part of it. Cancer is a fatal disease, unless you do something about it. We don't have the option of doing nothing and continuing to live. So we have to choose: Will I face it, will I fight it, or will I just die? If I strike back, there's a chance I'll have more life in this body, but there's no guarantee.

One way or the other I have to face the fact, *really* face it, that my days are limited. What will I do with them?

In days gone by, when a young man was trying to capture the affections of a young woman, it was said that he was "paying attention to her." It's still a good phrase. When someone is romantically interested in another, she or he pays attention to that person and tries to attract attention in return. The problem is that so often after we have been successful and nabbed the object of our interest, we *stop* paying attention.

I once knew a married couple who lived in separate wings of their house. They drove separate cars and went to different movies. There didn't seem to be animosity between them, but they just didn't pay attention to each other. One day I asked the woman why she had married the man, since they seemed to have so little in common.

"Well," she said, "he just kept after me, and the only way I knew to get rid of him was to marry him."

It's easy enough to do that with life, to get rid of it by marrying it. Then we can go our separate way, live in the far room, stop paying attention.

Cancer forces us to look at life again, to notice the part of the playing field we can't see. It gives us the opportunity to look at all the unlovely things about ourselves that we've gotten so used to that we do nothing about them. It gives us a chance to get our lives into shape.

I suspect folks get tired of hearing me say this, but I'll try it again anyway: I think I've lived more in the few months since I got cancer than I did in all the years before. I'm more aware of life, have better focus, experience each moment. I'm paying attention, and that lets me separate the wheat from the chaff.

Now that I have cancer, I'm thankful.

. . . *I'm vulnerable.*

AND I WANT TO take advantage of that vulnerability. I want to keep on being the new me.

Maybe I'll slide back with time. Perhaps my footprints on the sands of time won't be so crisp, so nicely edged, but instead will show the crumbling pattern of one who slips back with each step almost as far as he strides. Maybe I'll go back to shaking hands instead of hugging. Maybe I'll fall back to choking off the tears instead of letting them flow. Maybe I'll want to be "strong" again instead of open.

I don't want to backslide. I don't want to wall off instead of weep out, but I know it can happen. When my chemotherapy is over, and the cards and letters stop, and I have passed my five-year test and can eat colored food again, what happens if I become the old, "strong" me again?

"Strong" isn't bad. It isn't everything, either.

I like the new me, who weeps to see the little neighbor girl ride her bright pink bike, just because a healthy child in motion is such a beautiful sight.

I like the me who surprises men in gray suits with a big hug. It's a wonderful sight, two men in pinstripes, trying to figure out what to do with their briefcases while they attempt a hug—good laughter therapy if nothing else.

I like the me who talks to trees to let them know how well they are doing and how good they are looking.

I like the me who sings prayers, and laughs at silliness, and hopes all the time, without even knowing it, because it's so much a part of me.

I like the me who wakes up in the morning feeling joyful that there is so much to do instead of burdened because there is so much to do.

I like the me who welcomes pain as a friend because it reminds me that I am alive.

I like the me who isn't bothered by the chaos of my desk but covers it over with the sure knowledge of what is important and what is not.

I like the me who trusts the spirit more than the calendar and date books and lists and planners.

I've always had the cool, silent, determined courage of strength. Now I have the warm, bubbling, winging courage of weakness as well.

So I pray, "Let me grow, in both health and illness, into the new me. Let me be worthy of the new me. Let me be thankful for the old me—for the old me was a gift, too—but keep me vulnerable. Let every part of me move toward the whole me."

Now that I have cancer, I'm vulnerable, and scared, and glad.

. . . I have permission to pay attention to myself.

IT SEEMS THAT SOME folks pay attention to nothing else. Their lives are bordered on the north, south, east, and west by self, and that's all. They remind me of the man who prayed thus: "Bless me and my wife, our son, John, and his wife; us four and no more. Amen."

Most of us who get cancer aren't like that. We're pretty good people. We work hard. We feel guilty if we don't get things done. We blame ourselves if things go wrong. We feel that we have to make the world a better place. We're embarrassed if we're not making a difference. For people like us, any attention at all to our selves is selfishness.

Besides, we really are busy. We have jobs and families and friends and organizations. The whole world conspires to jam us in traffic and never to be there when we telephone and to get in line in front of us in the supermarket. There's just no time for self! We've got cars that are past their oil change mileage and toilets that are fighting back and children who are tugging at our legs. Even in the spare moments when we look wistfully toward the unread books and recall the times we prayed or meditated, there's no time to follow up.

So we've become machines instead of people, robots rather than persons, lists instead of lovers, date books rather than selves.

Now, however, there's a clearing in the forest. It's burnt over harshly, down to the stubble, but it's still a clearing. It gives me a chance to see with a wider view, a vision of the sky.

Now it's okay for me to take the time to visualize, to pray, to read, to nap, to sit, to stare, to meditate—to be.

A man dies and we hear someone ask, "What was he worth?"

"Oh, probably half a million," someone answers. Half a million what? Embraces? Prayers? Loves? Kindnesses? Sunsets? Bird songs? Walks? Meals with friends? "Of course not! Half a million *dollars!*" Is that all someone is worth? Dollars? If it's dollars, then it doesn't make any difference whether it's five or five billion. The same is true with all the other events and activities by which we usually measure worth. Did she make vice president? So what? Was he the star? Big deal. A forty-year pin? Big whoop!

It's not what you *do* but what you *are!* That's where this business of self comes in. My life has meaning not because I'm acceptable but because I'm accepted, not because I'm lovable but because I'm loved. I'm a part of life, a child of God. I *am!* Whether in this life or some other life, I *am.* I'm not a statistical summary—worked thirty years, married once, fathered two, made some bucks, watched some TV.

So now that I have cancer, it's okay just to be. Somehow I have permission from myself and the rest of the world to concentrate on this self, in order to get well. In the process, I have a chance not just to get cured but to get whole, to be who I'm meant to be.

Now that I have cancer, I have permission to pay
attention to myself.

. . . I live in shared space.

I SIT IN THIS shared space, in the waiting room of the cancer center, with people I have never seen before and may never see again. As I read their faces, though, I know we'll be forever in the same space, together.

Some of these faces simply stare into the middle distance, as though the space were empty. Some have eyes that I can see, but I know that they are staring into inner space. I can tell which is which, but I'm not sure just how I know the difference.

An old lady is eating a doughnut. A large plastic bag, cracked with age and cheapness, sits on the floor beside her chair; it is full of flowers. Her hair is pinned to her head with barrettes, but it's escaping in little wisps of gray—the color of memory. She's stuck into an ancient green pantsuit, twenty years out of fashion. Her face sags with an infinite sadness. One eye is clouded, as though it remembers only milkweed but remembers it well. The doughnut looks very small in her large and rough hands. They look like hands that have done the work they had to do. Because of that, they are beautiful.

It is clear that the doughnut is the highlight of her day. She takes tiny bites; it lasts longer that way. She holds each wee bite in her mouth, not chewing, letting it dissolve in a slow mirth on her tongue. Every bite is both a memory and a hope.

The tall, handsome man across from her uncoils and saunters to the doughnut table. He plucks one casually, rolls back to his seat. He looks like Rock Hudson doing a John Wayne imitation. He's draped in a new tweed Western suit, above shiny, two-tone cowboy boots. A bolo tie graces the front of his striped shirt. His fifty-dollar haircut insists that each strand keep the peace. His cowboy hat sits importantly in a place of honor in the chair next to him, trying to call attention away from the body he is trying to hide. He eats the doughnut as though he has no place to go, no past, and no future down inside him.

The man and woman with the gray hair look alike. Their glasses, their clothes, their hairstyles, the way they cross their legs, even the shapes of their bodies, match. They have been together for a long time. They share a doughnut, passing it back and forth, each taking a precise bite, no larger or smaller than the other. If I could see them kiss, I would see the lines of their cheeks match, flow together, groove into each other, so I could not tell where one begins and the other ends.

We share this room, this box of doughnuts, this space, although not by choice. This is a space of both despair and hope, fear and faith, anxiety and love. It is our space, together. I'm glad we share the space and the doughnuts and the hope.

I wonder what the other faces here read when they look toward me. Will they tell at the dinner table about the strange bald man who watched and wrote? Do they notice that I cut my doughnut in half, eat one side, then the other? Do they read that as a man divided, not whole? If so, they are right. But they also see a man whose eyes are wet with tears of solidarity as he watches the other doughnut eaters in this shared space. Because of that, next time they'll see a man without a knife.

Now that I have cancer, I live in shared space.

8. WHEN IT'S TIME FOR NEW THINKING

(ATTITUDE ADJUSTMENT)

Now that I have cancer . . .

. . . *It's a touching time.*

MY FRIEND BILL CAME to see me, a week after I was out of the hospital. He drove a hundred miles each way to spend an hour with me. We've been friends for almost thirty years. Between us we've had three wives and seven children. We don't see each other often, but we don't need to; our friendship is always still there. Bill's first wife left him ten years ago. Just told him one day she was leaving. No previous symptoms, even in retrospect. Just like my cancer. We share that kind of surprised grieving—he in his first marriage, me in my body.

When he was ready to leave, he sat on the sofa beside me and put his arm around me. I held on to his leg, like a little boy might wrap his arm around a father's knee. We prayed together. He told me he loved me. I tried to tell him I loved him, too, but I couldn't get it out. I believe he understood, though. Other than shaking hands, I think that's the first time we've touched, in thirty years.

Now that I have cancer, there seems to be an unspoken word of permission for people to touch me, for me to touch them. It's funny, that a broken body should somehow be more touchable than one that's whole. Or am I more touchable because my spirit is broken? "The sacrifice acceptable to God is a broken spirit; a broken and a contrite heart, O God, you will not despise" (Psalm 51:17). It is interesting that in all the stories of Jesus, there is only one instance of anyone touching him while he was alive in the body. He, of course, touched many: a leper, a hand to raise Simon's mother-in-law or Jairus's daughter up from beds of illness and death, deaf ears, blind eyes, the feet of the disciples, children. The woman with the hemorrhage reached only as far as the hem of his robe. The woman who broke the alabaster jar of ointment on his feet wiped it off with her hair—no touch. The only time anyone reached out to touch Jesus was to betray him, Judas with a kiss, the authorities of his own faith and people with a slap.

Maybe that's why "doubting" Thomas insisted on his famous touch-and-feel session after the crucifixion. Perhaps he was really "knowing" Thomas. Because no one had touched Jesus while he was alive, Thomas knew the real proof of the resurrection was that he could be touched, his body was broken. It's only after the breaking of crucifixion that resurrection, the touching time, comes.

Somehow we seem able to touch one another in our brokenness in ways we never can in wholeness. God likes to use broken things: broken bread, broken ointment jars, broken bodies, even relationships broken with a kiss.

My body and my spirit have been broken by cancer.
That means I can touch and be touched. I'm thankful
for the cancer.

. . . I listen to myself.

I LISTEN TO THE world around me, but I also listen to the world inside me. I listen to myself.

Most of us go through life without listening to ourselves, our own bodies and spirits. Therefore, we never know what we need, so we never get what we need.

Many of us are taught early on to be quiet about our own needs. You'd think that being quiet would lead to good listening, but it doesn't. It seems to work the other way around. The quieter we become, the harder it is to hear.

Sometimes our parents don't respond to our cries as infants, don't hold us, don't let us feel their love. We learn that there is no point in asking, so we shut up, quite completely. We shut ourselves up in cells of silence. Often we are rewarded for our quiet, are called good girls and boys because we shut ourselves up. We become proud that we never tell anyone what we need. We are silent, and we equate that with strength. We stop listening to the night cries of our souls because we'll never tell anyone what we hear anyway.

Others of us silence ourselves with our own voices. We talk incessantly, tell anyone about our problems, whine constantly, curse the day we were born and every other day as well. We prattle on just to hear our own sounds because they remind us that we still exist. Those around us get tired and stop listening. We get bored, too, and quit listening to ourselves. As Dylan Thomas remarked, "Someone is boring me. I think it's me." After all, we've heard it hundreds of times.

Our credo is found in a conversation you can hear any day in any small town post office: "How ya doin'?"

"Can't complain."

"Wouldn't do any good, anyhow."

Since it won't do any good, we don't bother to learn what there is to complain about, to listen to learn what our own needs are.

Now, though, I listen. Not so I can complain to others, or even to myself, but so I know who I am, so I can take control of my own life rather than leaving me shut up in some cell of silence. I have to know what I need, even if no one else does, because I am the one who has responsibility for taking care of this self. If I don't accept that responsibility, I'll have no self to be responsible for anything else.

"Fool, said I, you do not know / Silence like a cancer grows." Those are lines from Simon and Garfunkel's hit song "The Sounds of Silence." Silence grows like a cancer, and cancer grows in the silence. Not the silence of no sound but the silence of no listening. If we don't listen to ourselves, we can't listen to others, either.

There's a story about a piece of marble in Florence, Italy. All the sculptors rejected it because it was so ugly. Then Michelangelo came along one day and saw David trying to get out of it. Hence came one of the greatest pieces of art of all time. I suspect that Michelangelo listened not only to the cries of David, calling for freedom from the marble, but to himself as well.

I heard of an old man whose family asked him, in disgust, why he talked to himself all the time. "Why, because I like to hear what I have to say," he replied. It's a pretty good reason and a pretty good thing to do.

I certainly haven't given up on listening to my doctors and my friends and my family. But I listen to myself as well. My body and my spirit are telling me what I need. It's really okay to trust what I hear.

Now that I have cancer, I listen to myself.

. . . *I go slow.*

EVER SO SLOW. (I know it's not grammatical, but I like the sound of it, don't you?) Going slow is a luxury in our world. It's also a gift from cancer.

I've aged twenty years in five months. I hope to get twenty years younger in another eight months, when my chemo is over, but in the meantime, I'm a much older, slower guy.

That has some advantages. I'm more empathetic with older people than I used to be. I come up behind some slow mover in the oatmeal aisle and I don't dash around her as I used to, with a huff and a puff, showing off my young legs and eager lungs. So what if she has the aisle blocked with a prairie schooner that contains two small plain yogurts and a carrot? It's important to stand there and read all the cereal labels, to see how many grams of fat lurk in each brand. Now I might even linger a bit and point out to her that I like Uncle Ted's in the plain white box best because it has fewer preservatives than Nature's Normal All Natural, the one with the eight-color picture of a golden sun rising over a field of herbicides. (You just can't trust cereal box pictures, unless the picture is of Michael Jordan, of course.)

One reason I don't hurry around the other shoppers, I must admit, is that I can't. When you are aging a year per day, you slow down in a hurry. Besides that, my immune system is depressed by the chemotherapy, and I'm on a blood thinner because of the Groshong catheter in my chest, so I have to avoid infection and cuts with the vigilance of a long-tailed cat in a room full of rocking chairs.

Cancer is a natural slowing agent, and filmmakers have always understood that it's in slow motion that we learn what's truly important.

In this slow time, I am learning to be patient. I don't try to do several things at once. I concentrate. I do it well (as well as I can, at least), and I do it slowly, whatever "it" is. That slow motion is a reminder to myself that getting well is a lifelong process, regardless of how long or how short the life is. The living is in the process, not just in the result. It is important to experience each moment, not just the end.

Take writing this meditation, for example. Dorothy Parker used to say, "I hate writing, but I love having written." I was like that. I rushed through everything I did so I could mark it off the list and go on to the next line. I missed most of my life, because we live mainly in the "writing" and not in the "having written." So it's tempting to me to get this meditation done, to hurry on to the next one. After all, I have a lot to say, and I don't know how much time I have in which to say it. Isn't that reason enough to rush?

While I'm doing it, couldn't I also pray for those who will read it, and make a mental notation of where I have to be this afternoon while I'm writing and praying? Wouldn't that make the most of my limited time?

Whoa, there. Slow down. No one really does three things at once. We just think we do. Actually we switch from task to task with great speed and frequency. But the switching takes time, a nanosecond, regardless of how nimble we are at it. By doing but one thing at a time, concentrating on it, then switching to the next one, we actually save time, as well as wear and tear on our mindbody.

"Having written" is just a small fraction of life. I figure that even if cancer ends my days early, I'll actually get more living in than I would have with my precancer approach because I'm experiencing the "writing," too.

Now that I have cancer, I go slow.

. . . *I say "I love you."*

OH, I'VE WRITTEN IT on paper once in a while before cancer. I've even said the words occasionally. To the dog when we are out on a walk alone. To my wife when no one else is around. To my daughters on their birthdays. I think I even said it to my parents once. I'm quite open about saying I love the Cincinnati Reds and chocolate mint ice cream and Tony Hillerman novels, although I've never actually said it to a first baseman or a dish of ice cream or my copy of *Talking God*.

I know I scare some folks now. They think I've stopped short of the top floor. "Why does this bald man say he loves me?" they ask themselves. "Rational people just don't run around saying that all the time."

Well, having cancer knocks out a lot of rationality and leaves room for love to move in.

I know saying "I love you" can be very cheap. A movie star goes on a talk show and says to the host she just met, "I love you, daahling." Yes, it's hard to believe it means much. A man says it to a woman in the heat of lust so he can get "satisfied," without giving it much, if any, thought; it's just a means to an end. A child wails it to a parent to escape a spanking. A mother says it to pour guilt on your head at what you have, or haven't, done.

So many folks in our time cannot say it at all, however. Young couples talk about "the L word"; they can't even speak "love" out loud, for fear of commitment.

In Charles Schulz's *Peanuts* cartoon strip, Lucy is constantly trying to get Schroeder to fall in love with her. One day, disgusted with his lack of response, she asks Schroeder whether he even knows what love is. He immediately recites the dictionary definition of the word. With a scowl on her face, she says, "On paper, he's great."

We have a lot of paper definitions of love, a lot of songs and poems about it. It's not real, though, until it becomes embodied, in a person.

Helen and I were once in a group of couples. Each person was given pencil and paper and told to write his or her definition of love, without consulting anyone else. Then the leader had each person in turn read out his or her definition. This was a group of highly educated and intelligent people. As they read what they had written, each definition replete with beautiful and esoteric language, my heart began to fall. I could see by Helen's face that she felt the same way. When her turn came, she embarrassedly read out her definition of love: "John, and Mary Beth, and Katie, and Daddy, and Mother, and. . . . " She finished, and it was my turn. I read my definition: "Helen, and Mary Beth, and Katie, and Mother and Dad, and Uncle Ted and Aunt Nora."

We sat in silence. Then a strange thing happened. The other people in the group grabbed new sheets of paper and began to write lists of names.

Love is in relationships, self to self, body to body, spirit to spirit, or it does not exist at all.

I don't know why we have so much trouble saying "I love you," but I know cancer patients can get away with a lot that "normal" people can't, so here's what I propose: Say "I love you" all the time. To everyone: to the man or woman in blue who's giving you a ticket, to the discount store checkout girl who took so long you missed lunch, to the waitress who mixed up your order, to your teacher or boss or secretary. Then maybe we can say it also to the folks its really hard to say it to: husband or wife, children, parents, friends.

Now that I have cancer, I'd rather take the chance of saying "I love you" once too often than once too little, wouldn't you?

By the way, I love you.

. . . *I don't sweat the small stuff.*

I KNOW A WOMAN who has a plaque on the wall behind her desk. In large letters, it says: "DON'T SWEAT THE SMALL STUFF!" In smaller letters below, it says, "It's all small stuff."

The saying is half right. The small stuff isn't worth sweating. We spend so much time sweating and fretting and regretting about little things that don't matter. But it's not *all* small stuff. The small stuff is what my colleague and cancer friend Jean Cramer-Heuerman calls "ants around the ankles." It seems to me that there's a difference between the ants around the ankles, which aren't worth the sweat, and the details of life, which really are worthy of attention.

One of the things that impresses me most about Jesus is that he paid attention to the details but didn't sweat the small stuff. Remember Jairus's daughter? Everyone thought she was dead forever. Jesus took her by the hand and said, "Little girl, get up." She did, and the entire household was so overwhelmed by joy that they danced and shouted and whooped. They forgot Tabitha, the little girl. It was Jesus who said, "Look, she's surely hungry by now. Give her something to eat. A piece of fish would be nice."

A piece of fish? What a mundane thing. How could anyone think of a piece of fish when they had just seen someone raised from the dead? How could someone claiming his mission was saving the whole world be concerned with such a little thing? It was a detail, but to the little girl, and to Jesus, it wasn't small stuff.

I think the distinction is this: The details make a difference in people's lives, including my own. Paying attention to the details feeds someone. The small stuff doesn't feed anyone. In fact, it detracts and subtracts from the store of the world's love.

My problem is that so often I get the details and the small stuff mixed up. I can't tell the difference.

I get so worked up about remembering which telephone calls I need to make, and what to say in a particular letter, and whether anyone will get a certain room open in time for a meeting, that those ants around the ankles take over my life. They eat the whole picnic.

Sure, I have an organizational method. I have places I write these things down—many places! I even set my wrist alarm to remind me when it's time to do one of them. However, the method itself begins to contribute to my sweating of the small stuff.

I become absorbed in how to be ever more efficient. It's like trying not to think of a polar bear. I begin to think about small stuff done and undone as I run, when I pray, as I try to fall asleep at night. The small stuff is like water that seeps into a package of rice; all of a sudden the rice begins to swell and the package breaks.

The world around us doesn't make it easy to give up sweating the small stuff. Many people put a lot of pressure on us to make sure we get small stuff done. One of the reasons the world is in such bad shape is that we spend so much effort on the small stuff. It uses up all our energy. There's none left to use on the details, the details that get people fed.

It's not easy to make the distinction between small stuff and details, between ants and the picnic. For instance, what about doing the dishes? That's one of my jobs. Helen cooks and I clean up. It's a good arrangement since I have neither the creativity nor patience for cooking. Isn't washing dishes small stuff, though? No, because it makes cooking and eating possible. It becomes small stuff if I spend more than five seconds thinking about it, if I develop a computer program to tell me when and how to wash dishes. One clue that some part of life has become small stuff is when you can't break away from it, when the ants are gnawing at your ankles all the time.

You're sweating the small stuff if you're thinking about it at a time you can't do anything about it. If you're caught in a traffic jam, or waiting for a long train to cross, or imprisoned in a grocery line with a cashier who can't figure out how to scan Spam, there's no point in sweating it. You can't do anything about it. If you're at home, why think about something that needs attention at work? If you're at work, you can't be doing the dishes at home. If there's no solution, there's no problem.

There's so little time, even if I get well and live forty more years. There's no time to sweat the small stuff.

The ants are still gnawing, but I'm getting better at ignoring them. That's a gift from cancer.

Now that I have cancer, I don't sweat the small stuff.

. . . I live in the now.

RIGHT NOW. TODAY. THAT'S all. Because that's all there is. As one little boy is reported to have said, "There's tomorrow and today, so why can't there be a 'tonow'?"

I feel this, but I'm not sure I can explain it. I'll put it as simply as I can: What *eternity* means is that all of life is telescoped, from the past and the future, into this one present moment.

Looked at from one direction, there is no now at all. As soon as I have typed these words, they are already in the past. The ones that are yet to come are in the future. What we call the present is simply a razor-thin dividing line that keeps past and future apart.

When that divider is removed, however, and past and future run together, there is only now. I think cancer somehow removes the dividing line between past and future. When the divider is in place, there is no now at all. When it is gone, there is only now.

I've always been a person who enjoyed both past and future. I like remembering, and I like anticipating.

I recall with great pleasure the first time I met my wife. I can even remember what she was wearing. She had on a blouse, or a sweater, and a skirt, and some shoes. The clothes had colors, like green or brown. She also had hair. And she says I never notice anything!

I love remembering how my now-grown daughters looked when they were little girls, and how they used to push me off the sofa when I tried to take a nap after supper. I recall my grandmother and my first car and going to see the Reds play and marching into Montgomery with Martin Luther King Jr. I like living in the past; it's a good place.

The future is a good place, too. I've had the pleasure of anticipating all the things I've just remembered: our wedding day, and how the little girls would look when they grew up, and a Reds World Series victory. I look forward still—to seeing this book published, and going to support group tonight, and what heaven will be like. (I'm not too anxious to find out about the other place!) I like living in the future.

Somehow, though, as I live with cancer, the future and the past are both with me all the time. Remembrance and anticipation are both more real because they are both present, in the eternal now. The division between past and present isn't there anymore. I'm the sum total of everything I've ever been and all that I shall ever be. I used to be a library, full of many books, filled with many stories. Now I'm just one book with one page, but the whole story is right there.

I heard a tale that supposedly took place in the dry section of Nebraska. One farmer asked another why his pigs were so much fatter.

"We pole them," he was told.

"What's that?"

"When it's dry and there's nothing on the ground for them to eat, we tie them to a fifteen-foot pole and hold them up in the oak trees so they can eat the acorns."

"Doesn't that take a lot of time?"

"Hell, time don't mean nothin' to a hog!"

I'm beginning to understand that story, which worries me a little since it means I'm beginning to think like a hog! Time "don't mean nothin'" because it doesn't exist.

Albert Einstein, when asked to explain his theory of relativity, said, "An hour seems like a minute in the arms of one's beloved. A minute seems like an hour in the chair of one's dentist."

In the arms of God, there is no time. There is only love. That's what we call eternity, not endless time, but endless love. If you have love, you have all the time in the world right now.

Now that I have cancer, I live in the now.

. . . *I'm on vacation.*

IT'S A VERY STRANGE vacation, like none I've ever experienced before, but still, cancer is a vacation. My friend and colleague Jean Cramer-Heuerman, who also has cancer, understands this. She says we should write essays titled, "What I did on my cancer vacation." Well, here's mine.

I'm on vacation from a lot of stuff I used to consider so important that I just could not get away from it. Committee meetings. Piles of unread old newspapers and magazines. Unpruned bushes. Unpoisoned dandelions. Courtesy calls on people I don't like. (A "love" call on someone I don't like is different.) Getting all my Christmas cards in the mail on time—whatever "on time" is. Keeping records so I'll know tomorrow what I didn't do today, so I can keep feeling guilty about it. No guilt and no judgment—now there's a vacation!

I heard about a man who visited from church to church. He was looking for one where he would fit in. He slipped into the back pew of a new congregation a little late one day, after the opening hymn and just in time for the confession. He heard the people intoning, "I have done those things I ought not to have done, and I have left undone those things I ought to have done." He breathed a sigh of relief. "My kind of people at last," he said.

My kind of people, too, until now, when I have cancer.

I'm on vacation from all that guilt. Maybe it will come back someday, but I hope not. I like the vacation too much.

What is a vacation, anyway? It's a time away from the regular routine, usually in a different, maybe even exotic setting. Normal patterns are broken. There's time for doing something we choose rather than things that are required of us. We have a chance to get a different look at the world around us and the world inside us. Maybe that's why so many people don't enjoy vacations.

When I was "healthy," meaning strong in body and stupid in soul, a vacation always made me anxious to get back to work and routine and anxiety and justifying my existence. I had things to do, battles to win, worth to prove. Now that I have cancer, vacations make me want more vacation.

Don't get me wrong. I'm still working at my job, even during chemo week. Even during "reaction" week, which is worse. The vacation I'm on is a break from judgment, of others and of myself. I just spend my time lying on the beach of love, letting the waters of self-acceptance wash over me.

Come on down. Even if you're on 5-FU, this sun won't burn you, and the water's fine.

Now that I have cancer, I'm on vacation.

. . . *I'm getting things done.*

THEY ARE THINGS I'VE wanted to do for years, but I didn't have the time for them. There was no time because I did so much I didn't really want to do. Now I have less time, but I'm doing what I want to do. I'm finally a human being, instead of just a human doing.

I have less time, of course, because of cancer. Getting well is a full-time job, regardless of whether I'm alive or dead, what body I'm in, when the job is done. Surgery, visualization and meditation, chemo and its fatigue—they fill up minutes and hours and days.

I have more time, however, because I have cancer.

First it was recovering from surgery. Most days I just laid on the sofa, thinking and praying. But those were things I wanted to do then. No one expected me to do otherwise. When I had the energy to read, I read what I wanted, not what I had to plow through because of my job.

Then it was the suppression of my immune system by the chemotherapy. I was told to stay away from crowds and public places because I was especially vulnerable to germs and would have a hard time getting rid of them if they got a hold on me. Gradually I began to realize how much extra time I had because I was skipping the expected, whether it was a meeting or a movie.

It's not that I did bad or useless things before. The things other people expected me to do were not unreasonable. No one asked me to murder anybody, except, perhaps, me.

I still take out the garbage and wash the dishes and walk the dog. I still call on shut-ins (if they don't have germs) and preach at worship and work at the thousand other tasks that are my job. Someone needs to do those things, and I'm no better than anyone else just because I have cancer.

So what's the difference? If I have less time and more time because of cancer, how am I getting done those things I always wanted to do?

It's a matter of focus, I think. I simply see better what is loving and what is just doing, what is making the time fulfilled and what is just filling up the time. We have this incredible eagle-sized power of love, but we use it to hop around on the ground like one-winged sparrows.

I once lived in a city where I worked downtown. I was walking home after working quite late one night when I noticed that someone had flipped a cigarette butt up onto the canvas awning of a flower shop. It was slowly burning a hole into the fabric. The awning was too high for me to jump up to knock it off. There was no great danger, but I thought the fire could spread and ruin the awning. A phone booth stood on the corner. The fire department was just two blocks down the street. I telephoned the fire house and explained somewhat embarrassedly about the very small nonfire. I thought they might have someone walk down the street with a hand extinguisher.

Nothing happened for a while, and I was just about to walk on. Then suddenly fire sirens split the air. Trucks and cars roared out the big doors of the fire station—ladder trucks and snorkel trucks and an ambulance and even the chief's car! Because of one-way streets they blazed a six-block path through downtown. They arrived at the proper address, and the firefighters piled out of the trucks. They attached every conceivable hose to all the hydrants they could find. They ran in circles with axes and oxygen tanks.

The only problem was that they couldn't find the conflagration. By now people who lived in apartments above the buildings were hanging out the windows in their nightclothes. I wasn't about to point out the blaze, thus admitting to everyone just who had called this firefighting brigade into action.

Finally, in disgust, they began to pack up their equipment. Only one hose was left when the last firefighter saw the "flame." They quickly hauled the hose over to the front of the building, turned on the water, and blew the whole awning off the building and out into the street.

I think our lives are like that. We have the mighty equipment of love. With it we could put out all the fires of hate. But we use it on the little charred spots of our daily schedules instead of on the great conflagrations of our daily fears.

Using the time for love, that's the trick. If it's not loving, I just don't do it.

Now that I have cancer, I have time to get the loving things done because that's all I do.

. . . *I don't like cartoon shows on TV.*

WHILE STILL IN THE hospital, I started watching cartoon shows on TV in order to laugh. I need to laugh. I want to laugh. Laughter is healthy. When an anvil drops on Wile E. Coyote's head, though, I feel the pain. When Jerry blasts Tom with a cannon, I feel the hole.

So much of laughter is at someone else's expense. We want someone else to pay the price for our fun. We say we "split our sides laughing," but it was because someone else split his pants or head. So often our laughs are based on another's pain or humiliation.

That kind of laughter doesn't do me much good. It is antithetical to love. It is damaging instead of healing. Unfortunately, it's the kind of laughter that is taught to children from the cradle, through the cartoon shows.

Good laughter is a sign of the presence of God. It helps us get well. Bad laughter is a sign of the absence of love. It makes us sick. You see, it's love that heals. Laughter at someone else isn't love. It's just meanness. It may even do the laugher more harm than the one laughed at.

One of the most cheerful people I ever knew was Josephine Petry. Up to the day she died, of cancer, she always had a laugh in her holster, and she was the fastest draw in the county. After I had known Jo for a while, I was amazed to learn of the difficulties of her life. Before we had met her, she had spent six years nursing her husband in illness. In all that time, she never left their home, not once in six years.

I said, "Jo, how in the world could you survive a sentence like that? I know you loved Don and wanted to take care of him, but your home must have been a jail."

She smiled and replied, "Every day I found something beautiful to look at and something to laugh at."

I have no doubt that in spite of being shut in, Jo never watched the cartoon shows. She was always able to laugh at herself and, gently, at the foibles of the world.

A certain Roman Catholic cardinal lived a life of devout seriousness. Then he got sick. Everyone, including him, was sure he would die. His relatives came in and started dividing up his belongings. He lay in his sick bed, watching them, angry at their greed and insensitivity but unable to do anything about it. Then his pet monkey picked up his cardinal's hat, placed it on its own head, and began to admire itself in the mirror. It was so silly that the serious cardinal burst out in laughter and laughed himself right back into health and life.

That's healthy laughter—a good guffaw at ourselves and our own pretensions and our own failures, not the painful laughter that enjoys another's pain. Laughter is not a sure sign of the presence of either God or love, but God and love use laughter, healthy laughter, to put something beautiful into each day.

I'm much more sensitive to the pain of others now. I can't enjoy another's misery or humiliation or failure. I know what pain and fear are like. I also know how much fun it is to truly laugh with others, to laugh at myself, to laugh for the sheer joy of it.

Now that I have cancer, I don't like, or watch, the cartoon shows, but I'll be glad to have you laugh at me, with me.

. . . *I clean out drawers.*

AND FILES, AND BOXES, and shelves, and piles of stuff in the corner, and so on.

My first oncologist must be a football referee on his days off. He wanted to tell me how much time I had left in the game. "It'll be over in a year or two."

One of my first thoughts was, "I've got to get rid of my stuff." I have nineteen file drawers of notes and articles and clippings and letters and photographs and ideas. My boards and bricks host a thousand books, or maybe two or three thousand; I lost track a long time ago. I have boxes of old tests from college days and stacks of the high school newspaper I edited. I am surrounded by mountains of important magazines I'm saving to read when I get the time. Strong and hairy moving men have been known to weep upon seeing my stuff.

Can you sort through and get rid of fifty years of history and another fifty years of hopes in the brief span of one or two rotations of the earth around the sun? I was saving all that for retirement.

Then I learned from my next, continuing physician, Dr. Bernie Siegel, that the football officials might be wrong. What if I don't die in the predicted days? What if I get to write and speak and think and read for another ten or thirty years? Then my drawers and shelves would be empty, and I'd be like Mother Hubbard's poor dog.

If I die unsorted, though, my wife will have to deal with the stuff, which is hardly fair to her. She might not deal fairly with the stuff, either. I mean, she actually likes to clean and put things in order. Our daughters say that on her gravestone, it will read, in Prussian, "She got things done!" The only thing that has protected my stuff so far is that she is afraid of the alien life forms that inhabit my room.

So, a dilemma: to sort or not to sort, to toss or not to toss, to save or not to save.

I have decided the test is usefulness. Can I really use it? Does it have, or can it have, meaning? If it does, I keep it. If it doesn't, I toss it.

It's amazing how much I've dragged around, afraid to get rid of it when I really had no need for it. It's a good feeling to know that now I have control of the stuff instead of the stuff having control of me.

I've done that with my mind and spirit and body, too—hoarded up so much on the theory that I might need it someday. Then I just got used to having it around, until it clogged up all the space in my mind and spirit and body.

Now that I have cancer, I'm cleaning out the drawers—
of all *my rooms.*

. . . *I live in the open.*

NO, I DON'T MEAN I've taken my sleeping bag out under the stars. I'm certainly not out in the backyard barbecuing—have to watch that fat and smoke! I'm just not trying to hide anything anymore.

Of course, in some ways there is nothing I could hide. Once in the hospital a nurse was working on me. My wife stood down at the bottom of the bed, shifting around, trying to shield me from any passersby in the hall. I finally said, "Honey, don't worry about it. There's nothing I've got that everyone in the county hasn't seen by now."

That's not really what's out in the open now, though, especially since I got out of that backless gown. I'm talking about all the things we keep hidden about ourselves because we're afraid they're not acceptable, that people won't like us or respect us or—worst of all—love us, if they know the truth about us.

I've learned from cancer how dangerous secrecy is. Cancer hid itself in the dark places of my body and grew a tumor that I didn't even know was there. It wasn't until I got opened up that we could do something about that tumor.

So it is with the rest of life as well. Things hidden down inside grow and get bigger until they take over life and threaten it entirely. The word for this is *shame*. We are so ashamed of something that we keep it locked away, in the dark. Psychologists tell us that the difference between guilt and shame is that in guilt we think, "I did something bad." Guilt can be healthy sometimes because if we really did do something bad, guilt reminds us to go get forgiveness, to make the bad thing good. Shame, however, means "I *am* something bad." If I am something bad, there is no forgiveness, no way to make the bad good.

There is a healthy and legitimate sort of privacy, of course. There's no reason to speak out loud every thought we ever had, to tell the story of everything we ever did. Indeed, there are good reasons not to do so, such as not boring to death everyone around us.

We dare not use the healthy sense of privacy to cover up shame, however. It is appropriate to choose carefully where and when and with whom we are open, but if we are to get well, in the open we must live.

Through the years a number of members of Alcoholics Anonymous have done the fifth of their twelve steps with me. They sit down, sometimes with what looks like reams of notes, and simply pour out all the bad things they ever did, all the ways they hurt people, while under the influence of alcohol. Often they chose me for that role because I was safe. Some of them were people I never saw before or after. They didn't have to face me every day, knowing that I knew. It was good to choose someone like me. It could have been very hurtful had they shared that list of shame with a spouse or friend or co-worker or neighbor. It was necessary and important that they come out into the open with *someone,* though.

Most of us have addictions. They may not be to substances, such as alcohol or drugs or food or chocolate. They may be addictions to activities, such as sex or running. They may be negative activities, such as not eating. They may be to thought patterns: negativity, defensiveness, anger, unrealistic optimism, denial. Addictions are based on shame. They live in the dark. They make us sick, mentally and physically.

We need to take that fifth step, the step of honesty and openness, with someone appropriate. If our hidden places don't manifest themselves as addictions but we have the uneasy feeling that something is pushed down inside of us, it would be a good idea just to sit down with someone we trust and think that through, do some looking together to be sure no monsters can hide in the dark.

Getting well means getting honest.

Now that I have cancer, I live in the open.

9. WHEN IT'S TIME FOR NEW WAYS

(ACTION ADJUSTMENT)

Now that I have cancer . . .

. . . *I don't prepare.*

I JUST GO AHEAD and do it, whatever "it" is. I've stopped getting ready, stopped preparing. I figure all that time in my life I've spent getting ready is for what I'm supposed to be now.

If you've already read of my worries about cleaning out my boxes and file cabinets ("I clean out drawers," on page 128), you know that I have a fondness for keeping things. I'm not really a collector. It's just that I think this article or that scribbled note might be useful someday. I just want to be prepared.

Helen could easily toss all that stuff in a Dumpster if I weren't around to help, but I'm afraid that if everything gets thrown away unsorted, there might be lost a nugget or two that one of my daughters or a friend would like to have. There might even be a forgotten biscuit, since Waggs likes to give them as gifts and also hide them in case the great dog treat famine comes.

I remember reading a Halford Luccock column about a man who loved macaroons. He hid them all over his study—in books and file folders and piles of unread magazines. He was absentminded, so he promptly forgot where he put them. Then every once in a while, as he worked and rummaged in his piles of things precious enough to save, he would come across a "macaroon unaware." It was a serendipitous treat. I didn't want to die with any macaroons unaware not turned up.

So I started going through my files and piles, things that seemed so important in earlier days. I'm still sorting, because I'm enjoying it, and because I find I can throw things out now that I formerly needed for security, the way Linus clings to his blanket. There are things I have in my mind and heart now and no longer need to keep in a drawer.

Also, however, there comes a time when you have to stop getting ready and start doing. I've spent my first lifetime getting ready to live. Now, in my second lifetime, my cancer lifetime, I'm doing it.

I was also the type who not only had to keep stuff but had to have the proper equipment with me, too. I keep a ball cap and glove in the trunk of my car, just in case I come across a game that needs another player. I keep prayer cards there, too, in case I'm driving by a hospital and remember there's someone there I need to see, and I don't have my briefcase with me. Of course, that never happens because I *always* have my briefcase. What would I do if I got an idea and had no pen and paper?

Well, what I'm doing now. I'm in the doctor's examining room, waiting for him to work his way down the hall. There are no books or magazines in here—just tongue depressors and cotton balls. Here I am, with this great idea for a meditation about not preparing, and I don't have anything with me on which to write it. So I'm scribbling on the back of a prescription pad with a nurse-chewed pencil stub I found on one of those little tables. It works fine.

I'm not suggesting we should do away with insurance or never carry a comb or hankie. What I'm saying is that I'm learning to trust the spirit. Like Abraham finding the ram to sacrifice in place of Isaac, what we need will be at hand. It's probably safe to say that what we need isn't what we think we need; what we need is what we have.

I sometimes feel like I lived more in the first month or five after I learned I had cancer than in all my previous years put together. Those former years were good years, don't get me wrong. I don't regret them. It seems, though, that they were preparation for this time. I'm no longer preparing; the real thing is at hand. The time for storing nuts away for the winter is done; the time for eating them is here.

Now that I have cancer, I don't prepare; I just live.

. . . *I accept gifts.*

WHILE I'VE BEEN ON chemotherapy and had the Groshong catheter in my chest, my blood's been so thin I don't dare get a cut; it wouldn't heal. So John Mills cleans out my gutters. Bill Alexander mows my yard. I looked out the window one morning and there were Ross and Paulina Hunt, sitting on our front sidewalk, weeding the flower beds.

I remember one Christmas how Waggs, our dog, got caught up in the gift-giving spree. She went through her collection of bones and carefully left one for each member of the family. Mary Beth, who was a teenager at the time, didn't allow the dog into her room, so Waggs dropped her gift bone for Bethey just over the threshold. She put another in the middle of Katie's rug, one on the couch in my study, and yet another on Helen's side of our bed. It was systematic and thorough; there was no doubt what she was doing.

I'm sure it never occurred to Waggs that she should give anything to us because we had given to her, or that she might get something in return. I doubt that even the smartest of dogs, which Waggs really isn't, can think in such terms. She's never had any trouble asking (begging) for what she wants, without any thought for anything else. Somehow she just wanted to give gifts. It was an act of grace. Maybe that's why *dog* is *God* backward.

I've never been a good taker of gifts. A gift seems to leave the recipient in debt. A little bit of independence is forfeited when you accept a gift. The giver has a hold on you, even if there are no strings attached to it in a literal way. It may be no more than a word or telephone call or note of thanks that is required, but there's always something.

That's why we have so much trouble living by grace, whether

it's God's or someone else's. Grace is free, unmerited, no-strings-attached giving. Nothing forfeited to receive. No thanks necessary. It is so hard to believe that there can be a gift, a love, like that.

If we've been lucky, we've had someone in our lives who loved us that way. In the early stages it is often a grandparent. My grandmother never seemed to run my life, but her presence was always a blessing. She loved me and was proud of me and was willing for everyone to know it. I knew she'd love me regardless of what I did. Perhaps that's why I always wanted to do whatever would please her.

There are others who have reached out to me with grace-filled love, but I've never found it easy to take. Now, though, my resistance is down. There is so much I can't do for myself. I don't even have the energy to write thank-you notes. I'm so far in debt that I can never repay what others have done for me. I have to take, just because I need, without hope of paying back, making the scales even, being sure I never owe anyone anything.

Now that I have cancer, I'm learning not only the meaning but the reality of grace. I can receive a gift as just that, a gift. If cancer can bestow a blessing, then I'm receiving one: the gift of grace.

. . . *I don't keep score.*

I DON'T COUNT UP how many pages are left to read in the book. I don't count the seconds in my stretching-out exercises. I don't count the number of catches when I juggle. I don't figure up my mileage or my speed when I walk.

Love does not keep count. Love trusts the spirit and listens to the body. Love stays in the moment instead of comparing it to moments past. Love doesn't count on degrees and statistics and records and personal bests for its justification. Love reads because it's good to read, runs because it's good to run, stretches because it's good to stretch. Love does not keep score.

There's something within us that wants to keep score, that wants the records to prove where we've been and to point the way to where we might go. Masons have degrees, soldiers and police have ranks, academics have levels of professorships, students have grades, organizations have goals, businesses have sales charts. Baseball statisticians can tell us how many left-handed batters from Pennsylvania whose names begin with *W* have hit triples on July Fourth, and the last time it was done, and the odds of Walter William Winchell, a "triple" himself, hitting one this season.

In its own way, cancer is a record-keeping disease. There are times I have to take levamisole at home, outside the watch of the chemo nurses. (Levamisole is a sheepworm medicine. I appreciate it because not only is it getting rid of my cancer, it's also taking care of my lifelong fear of getting sheepworms!) I have a chart on which I record each levamisole dose. The nurses also want charts of diarrhea episodes and blood workups. My oncologist has a protocol that tells him what to do with me each month. In the early days of chemo, I kept a journal of my side effects—when they came, how severe they were, what happened.

As the chemo routine settled in, however, I began to realize the doctors and nurses weren't paying much attention to the records. They glanced at them and filed them, but then they put the emphasis on me. I wasn't just a history, a bunch of statistics. Once they were satisfied that nothing unusual was going on (as if everything about cancer isn't already unusual), they trusted their instincts, they trusted me, and they trusted the spirit. I stopped keeping my records and started listening to my body. It's a much better guide.

I'm not saying there's no place for history or records or statistics or scores. However, if you live by the statistics you die by the statistics. Living by the scoreboard means we have no other way of knowing whether we're doing okay. Living by the scoreboard indicates a life that has to be justified, a person who feels no right to be here unless she or he can show the world that record of production. That's the kind of person who is most likely to get cancer.

One thing we cancer patients know better than anyone, perhaps, is that you can't live life as a statistic and that statistics aren't a very reliable guide, either to the past or to the future. Your spiritual chances are much more important than your statistical chances. Keeping faith is more important than keeping score.

In the Rocking Chair Softball League (men over forty), we have a scorekeeper for the games, but she sits up in the stands and drinks Cokes with her friends. We usually don't know what the score is, even who won, until we're through playing, and we're not sure how reliable it is when we hear it. We've learned to play because it's fun to play, not because it's fun to have more runs than the other team. That kind of competition usually is not fun at all; it can be quite deadly.

Some will say, "What's the use of playing if you don't keep score, if you don't know who's ahead, if you don't know who won?" If you can play, you're ahead. If you played, you won. If all you know is the score, then you don't know the score.

Now that I have cancer, I don't keep score.

. . . I'm learning to be silly.

I MAKE UP SILLY songs and silly jokes. I use my time in silly ways, like juggling and working picture puzzles and building model airplanes. My imaging and visualizing and daydreaming are silly. I'm amazed by the world.

I didn't used to be silly. I was responsible. I was efficient. I was productive. I was serious—deadly serious.

What's the difference? Silliness is much more responsible and efficient and productive, that's the difference. Being serious is what's really silly.

I could do serious imaging about weighty matters, and people I don't like, and injustices that make me angry, and how the world is going to the dogs, if it hasn't already. I know how to do serious thinking about great problems for which I have no solutions.

I used to do that serious kind of visualizing. I imagined what I'd say if someone did something nasty. I argued with imaginary opponents about angry issues. I awfulized the breakdown of the car or the death of a friend. I anticipated getting caught in a traffic jam or in the slow line at the bank. I spent a lot of time being serious. It made me sick. Now that was really silly!

If we're silly, however, that means we're serious about being healthy. Norman Cousins found that when he laughed at the silliness of the Three Stooges, he began to get well. Serious medical people said that was silly. Wasn't that silly of them?

At the very least, silliness keeps me from thinking depressing thoughts, the sorts of images that lower the numbers of healthy agents in the body. Prayer is the same way. If I'm praying for myself or for others or for the world, even if the prayer is doing nothing else, it's using up my mind and energy so they can't see images and think thoughts that are negative, that will make me sick. Of course, some people think prayer is silly, too. They're right, of course. Prayer is silly, and silliness is prayer—and they're both good for us.

When children begin to have too good a time, adults say, "Now you're acting silly," or "Don't be silly!" I think adults are jealous of children. We aren't allowed to be silly, so we don't want them to be, either. "Get that silliness out of your head, child. Be serious. Be mature. Live a life of drudgery. Show how adult you are by getting sick and dying young."

I read the results of some medical research on two identical hospital wards with identical patients. The patients in one ward recovered better and faster than those in the other. The only variable was that the ward that did better had student nurses and the other one didn't. "Those silly, little student nurses," as one head nurse described them to me. They were silly enough to be enthusiastic, to believe their work made a difference, to trust that their patients really would get better.

Attitude makes a difference. Silliness is the best attitude. You get sick on serious, and you get well on silly.

Jesus said, "You can't enter the kingdom of heaven except as a child" (Mark 10:15 and Luke 18:17). How silly. All children do is play. Why does he think we spend our whole lifetimes trying to mature, to stop being like children? Children are silly. They don't understand how serious the business of life is.

Ah, the "business" of life. But life isn't a business, is it? It doesn't have a profit-and-loss sheet, a bottom line.

Life is given to us as a joy. Little children understand that. There's no business to what they do, they just do it. They look in wonder at the world about them and start laughing and roll down the hill.

I'm sure Jesus had childlikeness, not childishness, in mind. Child*ish*ness is when we think of no one but ourselves and our own immediate needs. It's a stage we need to grow out of if we're to live well with other people. Child*like*ness, however, is a stage we need to grow back into as adults, the stage when life is such a wonder and so much fun that we fall down laughing at it.

We want to be childish when we first hear that we have cancer. We're scared and hurt, and we can't think very far beyond ourselves. Getting well is moving from that childishness to childlikeness. Cancer helps us to get into heaven, because if we want to get well, we have to become like children again. Indeed, our task as adults, and especially as patients, is to become more perfect children.

It would *really* be silly not to be silly. No one gets well that way. It's never too late to have a happy childhood.

Now that I have cancer, I'm learning to be silly.

. . . I recycle everything.

IN THE CANCER CENTER where I get my treatments, there is a recycling bin in the lobby. "Why there?" the noncancered visitors wonder. "These people are fighting for their lives," they say. "These cancer patients won't be worried about the rain forests. They aren't concerned about tomorrow, because they might not have one. So why would they even bother to recycle?"

If you are a cancer person, I suspect you know why. Life in the world is too precious to waste. Every can and bottle is valuable, because every tree is important and every foot of land is holy.

Recycling is a symbol that something used, and even used up, can come around again in a new form, to give new life. We understand that.

Recycling is a way of acknowledging the interconnectedness of all life. In that way it is like prayer, which unites us with every creature through the source of love and creativity and constant renewing.

In the huge, extended McFarland–Pond family, until my generation there were only two people with cancer. Those two were people well into their eighties. Now, though, in my generation, I was struck by it at fifty-three. As I write this, my brother, only forty-five, has just undergone surgery and is starting chemotherapy and radiation. Why is this? Why does the incidence of cancer keep rising, until one out of every three people in America will hear that word applied to them?

There are many reasons, but one of them is that we've polluted our water and soil and air and spirit. We live now in a world made unfriendly by our own technology. It is a vivid reminder that the world is one. If there are cancer agents anywhere, physical or spiritual, none of us is safe. None of us can claim family health history or geographical place or status in the economic order as a barrier to cancer. We're in this polluted world together.

Recycling is a symbol of taking responsibility, not just for our own lives but for the life that we all share. It is also a way of expressing hope in the future.

Besides, we understand recycling because we are trying to do it with our own lives.

I once heard author Reuel Howe tell a story from his childhood. He grew up in the Pacific Northwest. His father lost his job and decided to homestead in the great forests. He took his wife and children and what possessions they had and trekked miles down an almost totally overgrown logging road to a rundown, leftover logging shack. Before they had been there one day, the shack caught fire in the early morning hours. Everything they had was destroyed.

Reuel was a teenager. He and his father walked back out of the woods and into town, where they were able to get tents and supplies. It took them all day. When they got back, they found that Reuel's mother had taken the little children and scouted around the site. They had found a rusty old tin can, some wild flowers, and a tree stump. The flowers were in the can. The can was on the stump. They were sitting around it, playing games at their new table, with its magnificent centerpiece.

She had taken a desperate situation and recycled it and made it good.

Now that I have cancer, I recycle everything. I just want to be in the habit. I want to recycle my life the way Reuel Howe's mother took a desperate situation and recycled it. Life and its parts are too precious to waste, even if I won't be a part of it in the days to come.

. . . *I worry about how much my treatment costs.*

NOT JUST WHAT IT costs me and my family directly, but our whole insurance group, and the entire health care system. It's easier to see my own costs, though, and to wonder what will happen to us if my insurance runs out. What if we have to take all our savings just to pay the extra expenses, like transportation and meals and sometimes an overnight stay?

They tell us not to worry, that anxiety suppresses the immune system and makes it more difficult to get well, but how do you not worry when the bills mount up, and you wonder whether you can keep on working or whether there will be a job for you when the treatments are over?

I have good insurance, but no insurance policy covers everything. Many patients have poor insurance or none at all. Not many of us have an extra hundred thousand or so buried in a tomato can in the backyard.

What do you do? Buy lottery tickets? Hope Ed McMahon comes through with one of those clearinghouse sweepstakes? Hit up your brother-in-law for a long-term loan?

Am I really worth this kind of money and this kind of worry? Is my life productive enough that everyone else should pay more for insurance because I'm the one who got sick? Should my family sacrifice new coats and vacations and cable TV so we can spend all our extra time and money on the trips to get my treatment and the extra medicines to counteract the effects of the chemotherapy?

Is anyone worth that kind of money? The pope? The president? Oprah? Geraldo? The director of Mickey Mouse at Disney World? Is there anyone we couldn't get along without and won't someday have to get along without?

When you look at it that way, I guess I'm as important as anyone else because I'm no more important than anyone else.

Each of us comes on stage and speaks our piece and goes off again. Some have better lines than others, but none of us built the stage in the first place. Nor did we assemble the audience. We can move the furniture around some, to make a path for the other actors or to make them stumble. We can ad lib or flub our lines. However, that is about as far as our power goes. We didn't write the play, and we have no idea how it will end.

It's not how much we produce in this life, how effective and efficient we are, that gives us a reason for being. Production is usually good, but not always. We've spent billions on nuclear and chemical and nerve weapons that are not good for anything. Efficiency is often good, but not always. The Nazis were terribly efficient in dealing death. The world would be a far better place if discount store clerks had been in charge of those concentration camps.

I'm here because I belong here. God put me here. I am a part of creation. If I can do some good, give something back, that's fine and dandy. But that's not why God put me here. God put me here to be a part of creation, not to do something to creation.

No part of the world is here because it is useful. It is here because it is here. That's true for rhinos and spiders and hawks as well as humans. If I say they have a right to be only as long as they don't get in the way of productivity and efficiency, only as long as they are "useful," then I have no complaint when the world wants to do away with me because I'm using rather than useful.

I still worry, but I only have to worry about where the money will come from, not about whether it's all right to spend my share on getting well. I don't mean to oversimplify. I know there are hard choices here, for me and for society. However, I also know that God has made each of us in creation as important as every other one. We belong here just because we belong to God and to one another.

Now that I have cancer, I belong. I think I have learned that from looking at the world around me.

. . . *I live in my body.*

MANY PEOPLE DON'T. I know, I've usually been one of them. I was formerly a brain that used a body. My body was a handy tool for getting my brain from place to place. I know a deep muscle therapist who says most of her clients want to drop their bodies off, let her work on them, then come back to pick them up. They don't even want to spend their spare time in their bodies, let alone live in them.

The body is our home, however. Our bodies are temples, but we usually treat them more like motels. The basic reason disease happens is that we don't live in our bodies. We do things to our bodies that we wouldn't do if we lived there.

I have a friend who says, "If you want to be well, come home. Inhabit your body."

This body home has an extensive communication system. There are many "I"s within me, and they are not just the characters that inhabit my brain. Emotions are not just in the brain but in the body as well. Every hurt we've ever experienced is stored somewhere in the body. There's a mind in every cell. Each cell is a microcosm of the whole. Indeed, Candace Pert, the chief of brain biochemistry at the National Institute for Mental Health, says, "the body is the outward manifestation of the mind."

Whenever one part of the body is abused or neglected, it tells the rest of the body about it, complaining of its treatment. All the other parts get upset, for unlike people, the "I"s of the body never forget that they are related, that they depend on one another, that if one gets sick they all might die.

Now I talk to my body, and I listen to it. I ask each part how it is doing, whether it has any complaints, if the rest of us can do anything for it. I lay hands on the parts that hurt, because that interconnected healing touch is one of the jobs of the hands. I ask the parts to get along together and work together. It's amazing how well my body responds to being treated like somebody.

To get well, we have to stop using our bodies as though they are tools and live in them, because they are homes.

I've come home to my body. Before, I always rushed through bathing, dressing, even eating. I always tried to do some useful work with my brain while I was also using my body, whether it was running or sitting or showering. Just doing something because it was necessary for my body never seemed to be adequate. I had to do something "productive" at the same time. I had to be efficient.

Now I don't try to forget about my body. If the body is doing something, I stay with it, go along for the ride, remain in the moment, see whether it likes it. I live in it, even at the times of pain.

The little child I hear in a room down the hall in the cancer center has the right idea. He's crying and screaming, "No shots anymore," over and over. Good for you, little fellow. You're living in that body, and you're letting it tell the world how it feels and what it needs. You'll get well faster. (Your parents and doctor might go crazy faster, too, but that's their problem.) I'm not as good at living in my body yet as you are, but I'm working on it.

Many people are impressed with out-of-body experiences. I am, too, but I'm even more impressed by in-body experiences. Those are what you have when you live in your body. They help you get well.

Now that I have cancer, I live in my body.

. . . *I laugh.*

A LOT.

Although there have been days of worry and discouragement in my life, when I found it hard even to chuckle, I have always loved humor of any kind. Now, though, I go out looking for laughs with a net.

There are many reasons why we laugh. It's healthy. Norman Cousins tells us to. It's almost impossible not to sometimes.

Why do we laugh, though, when the humor is almost designed to scare us?

The doctor told the cancer patient, "You have six months to live." The patient replied, "But doc, I can't even pay your bill in six months." "In that case," says the doctor, "you have twelve months to live." Now why would we laugh at a joke like that? How can one laugh in the face of death?

Well, what else can you do in the face of death? Kim Wagler was my first oncology nurse. Her youthful energy and upbeat style and infectious laugh were as important to me as what she taught me about dealing with the disease and the chemotherapy. A few months later, she learned she had cancer herself, of the breast. "The gal with the great laugh," as she is known to all, found that black humor was very appealing to her in those early days of her diagnosis. She was the one who told me about the soap opera for cancer patients, *The Young and the Breastless.* Why would a joke like that make a breast cancer patient laugh?

Well, I think the answer is twofold. For one thing, it's just better than any of the alternatives. If you've only got six months, or twelve if the doctor is greedy, wouldn't you rather spend it with a laugh on your lips and a song in your heart than with a moan on your lips and quicksand in your heart?

For another thing, the serious side of cancer is just so scary. What will happen to us? Will we suffer in some terrible way? Will death be an end to all the good things we love so much? Thinking about those serious issues only makes things worse. The most likely result of worrying about suffering is suffering. Laughter may not keep us from bad things, but awfulizing won't keep us from bad things, either.

I have a friend who has been in a serious, responsible, important, seventy-hour-a-week job for several years. Before he took it he was known as one of the most humorous people around. We have always joked a lot together. I came across a funny magazine article that fit his job exactly, poking gentle fun at it. I sent the article to him, figuring he could use a laugh or two. He returned it with a very serious and somewhat antagonistic note that said, "I'm sending it back so you can give it to someone who might see the humor in it." I worry about him. I pray for him. I try to laugh about things for him, because his job has squeezed out of him the ability to laugh, especially at himself. The inability to laugh is the prelude to illness.

It's well known by now that laughter brings out the best in us, literally. A good belly laugh increases remarkably the levels of all the healing agents in the body. The old adage that laughter is the best medicine, or at least one of the best, has been scientifically proven.

I couldn't do belly laughs after my belly had been cut open from San Diego to Boston, so I had to make do with smiles and chuckles. Any laugh you can muster, especially when the pain is at its worst, is not only a strike in the healing lane but a laugh in the face of the devil.

Allen Klein publishes the *Whole Mirth Catalog*. He became a laughter collector while nursing his wife through her cancer, looking for anything that could bring a smile to her face. He made us laugh for a whole afternoon at an American Cancer Society seminar. I ordered a laughter cassette tape from the catalog. That's all it is: people laughing. When I feel down, I pop it in my boom-box and turn the volume up. People laugh all over the house. Pretty soon, I'm laughing, too. It feels so right.

Did you hear the one about. . . .

Now that I have cancer, I laugh—a lot.

. . . *I wear my best clothes, all the time.*

MY NEW "OUT OF Africa" hat. My brown boat shoes or snowy white Reeboks. My fashionable madras plaid shirt. My "prestressed" green casual coat, with the hood and wooden buttons.

This is a giant step for mankind, according to my wife and daughters. Before cancer I had two methods of choosing what to wear. The first was to take whatever came up next in the closet, regardless of color, cut, or style. The other was that if whatever came up next was too new—less than ten years old—I put it back at the far end of the rack, to be saved for a special occasion.

Well, the special occasion is here. Today is the most special occasion I can imagine. If I have a tomorrow, that will be a special occasion, too. There will never be a better time than right now. So today I'm wearing my new oatmeal pullover. If tomorrow comes, look for that ritzy new corduroy blazer. Look out, world; I live for fashion!

Not really, of course. I live for love. Wearing my best clothes is just a way of saying that right now is the time for love. I'm sure my mother loved me when she taught me to hold my good clothes back until that really special time came to wear them. After all, when I was growing up, I had only one "good" shirt, and only one pair of shoes, for all occasions. It was important to take care of what we had. Who knew when you would get something new?

These days I know more about my clothes than about how many days I'll have. Who knows how many times I'll get to wear my Cincinnati Reds baseball cap? No use waiting for the World Series. I'm a Reds fan today, and I want everyone to know it. I'm a life and love fan today, too, and I want everyone to know that. When you see me coming down the street, I want you to know that to this man, today is a special occasion.

One of the most poignant stories out of Vietnam was that the soldiers always ate the peaches from their C rations first so that if they got killed, they wouldn't have missed the best part of the meal. Perhaps that's where this saying came from: "Life is short, so eat dessert first."

Remember the story Jesus told about the wedding feast? (You can read about it in Matthew 22:13–14.) The king who threw the party discovered a guest who had not bothered to put on his wedding garment. It was an insult to the host, who had the man "thrown into outer darkness." "*This* is the day the Lord has made. Let us rejoice and be glad in it." Let's dress like we're glad. Put on your wedding garment. We're being called to the feast, the feast of the eternal now. There's no point in waiting for a better invitation, a more special occasion. We're invited to the party, right now.

Get out that new dress, sister. Put on that bright tie, brother. This is *the* special occasion. You figure you'll only get to wear it once? All the more special. Whoever gets it next will be pleased to have it, even more because you wore it.

Look for me in the Easter parade. I'll be wearing my Crocodile Dundee hat, a blue and red rugby shirt, and tan pants with cargo pockets.

Now that I have cancer, I wear my best clothes, all the time.

. . . *I listen to my body.*

OH, I ALWAYS DID that, of course. We all do, to some extent. Our bodies tell us things we have to listen to. We get tired and must lie down. A leg hurts so badly we limp. A stomach churns up so badly it turns you inside out. The throbbing head, the aching back, the pain in the neck, they all cry out for attention. They talk to us, and we are forced to respond.

However, our response often is just an attempt to get rid of the pain so we don't have to listen anymore to what that part is saying. We basically want to ignore our bodies, keep them quiet. Like children are so often told, "You are to be seen and not heard."

Now I try to listen, to hear what my body is telling me through its pain rather than just trying to shut it up. Disease is a message, not just about a pain that needs to be obliterated but about a life that needs to be healed.

Of course, the body does not want to hurt. It speaks to us through pain so we'll do something about what is causing the pain. I heard of a man whose life was so twisted that his friends said when he died he had to be screwed into the ground. That's an awful epitaph, isn't it? There was a man who didn't listen to his body.

I listen to the messages from my body, but I also listen to the body's witness, the statement the body is making about the nature of life. One witness of the body to life is the interconnectedness of it all.

When our daughters were still in preschool, I had a household accident. I had my index fingers stuck in the loops of a self-storing window screen, trying to raise it, when the heavy glass storm panel fell so quickly that I couldn't get my fingers out. It came down like a guillotine, smashing the ends of my fingers. The pain

156

was excruciating. I thought of all the cusswords I had ever heard, and none of them were even worth saying; they would have been so inadequate.

My fingers were flat and purple for weeks. I had to hold them straight up, above shoulder level, to ease the pressure on them. The girls sat around, clucking their sympathy, and one of them said, "Daddy *all* broke."

She was right, of course. Although only a tiny fraction of my total body was directly affected, I was all broke. My entire body shared in the pain. The whole body had to contribute to the healing. One part cannot be diseased without putting the complete body in harm's way.

Another witness of the body, clearly related to the connected nature of life, is love. Love, peace, and joy are emotions that heal the body. Hate, division, and resentment are emotions that destroy the body. Nature, at its core, is telling us what it wants, what we are made for, by the ways our bodies react. If we were supposed to be hateful grouches, our bodies would thrive on strife. They don't, though, do they? Our bodies get well on love and happiness.

The body's witness, to which I do best when I listen, is that we are made to relate to one another, to be connected, in love.

Some of my best friends, who bear with me through thick and thin (literally), who will tell me the truth, honestly, are the parts of my body. They tell me, "Hey, you're doing something, or not doing something, that makes us hurt. Let's get this straightened out."

Sometimes, of course, all I can do is apologize. Like when I'm taking chemo, and a whole chorus of voices comes up from my body that says, "What in the hell are you doing?" I explain that this is going to hurt right now but will make us all better in the long run. They accept that and say, "Oh, well that's okay then. We're glad to cooperate."

So we talk back and forth, but now that I have cancer I do more listening than talking. It's amazing how much you can learn when you listen to your friends.

Now that I have cancer, I listen to my body.

10. WHEN IT'S TIME TO SAY "NO"

(DEALING WITH OTHERS)

Now that I have cancer . . .

. . . *I've put my megaphone away.*

I'VE PUSHED IT TO the back of the closet, along with my brown and white saddle shoes, and my yellow sweater with the big smiley face on it. Sound familiar? You got it—a cheerleader no more!

A lot of people—friends, family members, folks we work with, just people we meet on the street—expect us to be cheerleaders when we have cancer. They want us to jump up in the air, yell "rah, rah, rah," claiming, "Everything is fine and dandily, we are winning, oh, so handily."

Well, I'm more likely to sink into a chair, mutter "raw, raw, raw," and grumble, "I feel like a total wreck, or second opinion, I feel like heck."

There's a *Peanuts* cartoon strip in which Charles Schulz has Linus telling Charlie Brown that he would like to be a prophet when he grows up. "That's nice," says Charlie Brown. "The problem is that prophets almost always turn out to be false prophets." "Maybe I could be a *sincere* false prophet," suggests Linus.

Sincerity! That's the mark of a cheerleader, isn't it? However, sincerity alone doesn't cut it. People can be quite sincere about things that are very bad. False prophets can be totally sincere, but they are still false.

Don't get me wrong. Some of my best friends are cheerleaders. Especially now. I need cheerleaders.

I love it when my friends tell me I'm still doing good work: "Two, four, six, eight! Who do we appreciate?"

I feel better immediately when my wife proclaims how much she loves me and how she never felt closer to me.

"He's a wonder! He's a dream! He's the captain of our team!"

I need to have a chemo nurse grab a big flag with my name on it and run three times around the treatment room screaming, "Push 'em back! Push 'em back! Farther! Farther!"

I cherish the hugs and pats and words of encouragement that come from all my cheerleaders. They lift me up on a cloud of love, and I can fly!

There are times when I've led the cheers for each of them, and times when I do now, but those cheers aren't about me. I need their cheers; they need my cheers. We get into trouble, though, if we expect one person to be the patient and the cheerleader, too. I can't lead the cheers for me.

What's healthful and wholesome for me is to be honest about how I feel, not to put on my yellow cords and white socks and claim everything is okay. It's unfair of anyone to expect dishonesty from me.

Imagine this: A runner comes into the stadium full of people at the end of a marathon. He looks up into the stands and sees thousands of people, all sitting on their hands. They say, "You're okay, aren't you? You're not feeling bad, are you? Please assure us you'll make it to the finish line just fine." But he *doesn't* feel good. It's been a long, hard, grueling race. Nonetheless, the runner waves and shouts and assures them everything is okay, and he's so out of breath everyone else in the race runs right on past while he drops to his knees.

Or imagine this: A runner comes into the stadium, barely able to keep those legs moving. Suddenly the crowd is on its feet, shouting, screaming, cheering. She's swept up in the adulation. A wave of energy comes down and picks her up and hurls her toward the victory line. She's not even aware of her feet touching the track. She reaches back and finds more breath in those depleted lungs. She knows she's a victor even if she falls on her face.

We can't be the cheerleader and the runner both. We need the cheers, but they must come from others. Our strength has to be put into the race itself.

Now that I have cancer, I'm the runner, not the cheerleader. That's okay.

. . . I don't do favors for friends.

WELL, NOT MANY, ANYWAY.

Dr. George F. Solomon says there is one simple question you can ask yourself to gauge your chances of long-term survival. "Would you do a favor you didn't really want to do for a friend who asked you to?" If you say "yes," there go your chances. That's because you fit what Dr. Lydia Temoshok calls the Type C coping style for cancer patients: compliance, conformity, self-sacrifice, denial of hostility or anger, and nonexpression of emotion. It's a pattern we learn in childhood. It's also a pattern that ought to serve us cancer patients well, it seems to me.

Why are all these doctors telling us we have an attitude problem when we are just trying to be nice? After all, we are supposed to keep an upbeat attitude. What better way to do it than to paint a smile on the old stiff upper lip? Shouldn't we shout a cheery "just fine" whenever anyone asks us how we are, regardless of how bad we feel? We don't want to be a burden to our families and friends. Maybe they won't like us anymore if they have to take our pain seriously.

One man in my community is lifted up by some folks around here as the ideal example of a cancer patient. "Dan just kept working right up to the day he died," they say. "You'd never even know he had cancer." They say that mostly when I take a day off from work. I have considered all this, however, and it occurs to me that Dan, as admirable as he was in many ways, is not a good model for me. Dan's dead.

I certainly understand that we are all going to die someday. I don't blame Dan for his death. If he wanted to work up to the day he died, that's okay. That was his choice, although I worry about some of the people who loved him. They may have felt neglected and left out by his decision.

I don't want to work up until the day I die, though. I don't want to smile and say everything is fine up until the day I die. I want to *live* up until the day I die! That may include some hours on the job, but many, it won't.

If saying "no" to doing favors is going to help me live, then I'm going to say "no." If telling people I feel miserable when I feel miserable is going to help me live, they are going to know I feel miserable. If getting mad at the world's injustice is going to help me live, then look for me on the picket lines. If breaking down and crying and telling the people I love how much I care about them is going to make me live, then get out the tissues and hankies. (It's interesting that we call that "breaking down," isn't it?)

I'm not afraid of dying (well, not much), but I don't want to be afraid of living, in all life's fullness, either. Many of us cancer patients are more afraid of living, in a new way that will help us, than we are of dying. We'll just slip away quietly; no one will ever know.

Certainly I haven't stopped doing things for folks. If someone asks me for a favor, and I can do it without detracting from my wellness, I'm glad to do it. It makes me feel good. But that's the trick, isn't it? I do it because I want to, not out of that old feeling of obligation. I'm not going to do any more favors with a smile on my face and a frown in my heart.

Now that I have cancer, I don't do favors. I only do wellness.

. . . *There's no one worse off than I am.*

NO, I DON'T BELIEVE that, but I say it to remind myself that each of us is unique, that we're not here just for comparison purposes. People always say that, don't they? "You can always find someone who's worse off than you are." I know that's true. I say it to myself all the time, but I resent it when others say it. They diminish me by treating my pain as insignificant unless it's worse than everyone else's. Is no one worthy of any sympathy unless she or he is the only one who is worse off than everyone else in the world?

I sit in the chemo treatment room. To my left is a teenaged boy, his clinch-jawed mother perched on the edge of a hard plastic chair beside him. They are both worse off than I am—he because he's so young, she because her child is ill. I'd much rather deal with my own cancer than know it is growing in one of my children. I sneak furtive glances at their faces, the blankness of his and the lines of hers, and I know that by comparison I am blessed.

Across the room, beside the aquarium, sits an old woman. The tiny orange and blue fish do their best to entertain her, but she doesn't even see them. Her eyes are open, but she's looking inward. Her only hair is a patch of scraggly brown, down low behind the left ear of her bullet head. Her swollen legs end in rundown house slippers. She is worse off than I am.

To my right is a pretty young woman, the mother of three. I remember her from the waiting room in earlier visits, before the cancer took her breast. She was wearing a red sweater then. Every man in the room looked at her more than once. Now she wears a loose smock and makes herself small as she hunches down in the chair. I still look at her more than once. She knows it is out of concern for her loss rather than appreciation for her curves, and she both appreciates and resents it. She's worse off than I am.

I scan the room. I pray for each of them in turn. I try to speak with my eyes, spirit to spirit, saying, "I've got a little extra strength today; take it, and use it." I do it because I know they're worse off.

If someone else walked in right now, however, and said to me, "Well, just look around you. You can always find someone worse off than you are," that boy and his mother, and the old woman, and the young mother would all stand up and shout, "Get out of here. He's here for the same reason we all are. Don't reduce any of us by comparing us one to another. Each of us is worse off."

We need to count our blessings, but not as a cover-up for our real problems or like a game of winners and losers, "My blessing pile is bigger than yours."

We who are being healed of cancer, even though we are not all being cured, know that we belong to one another. We understand one another in a way no one else can understand us.

Love us. Love us all, please. Just don't compare us.

Now that I have cancer, there's no one worse off than I am.

. . . *I have cancer.*

THAT'S HARD ENOUGH FOR me to believe and understand. It seems to be even harder for some other people. Not only do I have to deal with my own denial, I have to cope with theirs as well.

I'm very open about having cancer. I talk about it all the time, although I try not to say the same things to the same people. I'm trying, by being open, to pull the fangs of the beast that feeds on secrecy, that makes us afraid because it's hidden in the dark. I'm doing it both for myself and for others. Others don't always appreciate it, though. One way or another, they make it clear they'd be happier if I'd shut up and act like I just have a sprained toe.

Many people praise the patient who acts like nothing has changed as the ideal. They're saying, "I don't know how to deal with you now that you have cancer, so I want you to play along like you don't have it. Don't bother me with it, and I'll like you and praise you for your attitude."

That's a lot of pressure. Implied is the threat that if we don't go along with their denial of our cancer, they might just deny *us*. They might withdraw entirely and blame us for the new chasm between us, blame us for getting cancer. Whew!

Some folks actually do pull out. I know a cancer patient whose husband said, "I just can't handle this." He left. *He* couldn't handle it? What about her? It's easy to say she's better off without him, but we need our friends and family so much right now that we usually do what we must in order to hang on to them, even if that means acting like it just ain't so.

I heard of a man who had cancer for ten years and never told anyone in his family. He was a salesman, so he arranged to get chemotherapy treatments out of town while he was on his rounds. Once a year he went to the Mayo Clinic in Minnesota, but he told everyone he was going on a hunting trip. Was he just a private person? Or trying to protect his family? Or was he afraid of how they would react?

What should we do when family members and friends want us to go on like "normal"? Some patients are expected to wear a wig even at home, do the dishes even though they are so nauseated they can barely stand, arrange chemo schedules so they can still take the kids to piano lessons, or stay out of sight if they look sick.

Well, things are *not* the same, and if other people can't handle it, that's their problem! We're not doing such folks any good by accepting their denial, and we certainly aren't doing ourselves any good. I don't have the strength now to deal with other people's expectations. All my energy has to go into getting well, not acting like I'm not sick. I'm not going to die quietly so that after the funeral they can say, "Wasn't he good about it? He never bothered us at all."

Jesus had some similar problems with the Pharisees. John tells us about Jesus healing a man who was born blind. The Pharisees really preferred that the man remain blind. They saw Jesus' healing activity as a judgment on their unwholesomeness, which, of course, it was.

"Are we also blind?" they asked him. Jesus said to them, "If you were blind, you would have no guilt; but now that you say, 'We see,' your guilt remains" (John 9:40–41).

When we claim to have no illness, we cannot accept healing. When we allow others to push us into denial, we're letting them deny us life in the spirit, and quite possibly life in the body as well. I won't get well, in spirit or body, unless I first admit reality.

Now that I have *cancer, I* have *cancer. There! In your face, Pharisees!*

. . . Some people won't talk to me.

THEY DON'T EVEN WANT to see me, and I'm pretty good-looking for a beat-up old guy! I don't look much different. Hair's a little thinner. Lips get red and puffy after chemo. Eyes get sort of slitty, for the same reason. I've got an abdominal scar from L.A. to N.Y., but no one sees that. They don't see the pretty blue catheter in my chest, either. (My younger daughter, an avid Cincinnati Reds fan, took one look at it and said, "Oh, no; it's Dodger blue!")

They don't want to touch me, either. In the meditation called ". . . It's a touching time" (page 108), I tell of how cancer makes us more touchable to some folks because of our brokenness. That's not true for others. Are they afraid it's catching? Surely not; almost everyone knows better than that these days. But there's something about us cancer people that makes others afraid. One of the men in my support group told us of a man who actually got up from his booth in a fast-food restaurant and moved to the most remote one he could find when my friend sat down at the next table. It's strange how cancer makes us more touchable to some and less touchable to others.

These folks are like the three monkeys: See no cancer people, touch no cancer people, and, especially, talk to no cancer people.

Are they just afraid they'll say the wrong thing, like "You don't look too bad for a corpse"? Maybe; none of us wants to stick that smelly foot in our mouth.

However, I think it's mostly that I'm a walking (slowly, but still walking) reminder that "it" can happen to anyone.

Even them. Especially them. My very presence is a symbol of vulnerability. It's especially bad for those who knew me before, because I was always so strong, so healthy. Not a symptom of any kind. Then one day I had "it." If it can happen to me, it really can happen to anyone.

If I try to talk to them of death, even of pain or fear, they brush it off. "Oh, you are going to be fine," they say. If I persist, they don't say anything at all. They are gone as fast as a hamburger in a tiger cage. They cross the street when they see me coming.

I wish they would talk with me. They're missing something special. So am I.

I wonder whether Jesus felt that way. When he was tried, and found guilty, and nailed to a cross, all his best friends deserted him. Not only did they not want to talk to him or see him, they didn't even admit they knew him. That must have been very lonely.

So I do for those who won't talk to me what Jesus did on the cross for those who persecuted him. I pray for them. They won't talk to me, so I talk about them behind their backs, to God. God and I have entered into a conspiracy of love. The more those folks refuse to talk, the more we talk about them. We don't try to change them. We just love them. I still wish they would talk. It would be good for them. For me, too. But until they have ears and tongues, they are at least going to have prayers.

Better look back, you silent ones. Those sounds you hear are the wings of prayer. Gotcha!

Now that I have cancer, some people won't talk to me.

11. WHEN IT'S TIME TO SAY "YES"

(DEALING WITH OTHERS)

Now that I have cancer . . .

. . . *I worry about my wife.*

I'M SURE YOU WORRY about those who love you, too. We tell ourselves not to worry, that worry doesn't help anything. We go ahead and worry, anyway. It goes with the territory called love.

I worry about Helen's health; will concern for me make her sick, too? I worry about her future; what will happen to her if I die, or take too much care, or cost too much money? I worry about her peace of mind; how can she work and take care of me and face loss and still be the sane and wholesome person she's always been?

I think this cancer business is harder on her than it is on me. Sure, she's not the one who got cut open. She's not the one who hugs the porcelain fixture after chemo, or gets her eyes glued shut, or has feet too swollen to walk on. I'm the one who had the operation, who gets the chemo, who lives with the symptoms.

I'm not the only one who has to struggle through all these, day by day, however. In the way of love, she was cut open by the operation. The symptoms make her sick, too.

It's the difference between being the driver of a car and the front-seat passenger. Before seat belts we called that the suicide seat. It's still an apt name for the passenger on a cancer trip.

When an accident starts, you don't know how it will finish. The car fishtails on the ice and then begins to spin. You look down the road and see a truck coming. You steer with the spin and look for traction. You don't know whether you can keep it in your own lane, but you're doing your best. All that is what's happening on the driver's side.

In the passenger seat, all you know is that something is terribly wrong and you can't do anything about it. There is no steering wheel in your hands, no brake pedal beneath your foot, no gear shift or lights or horn that you can use. You can only pray and trust the driver.

It's the same on a cancer trip. The sudden spin starts, and you don't know how it will end. We patients have the wheel in our hands. We're scared. We're mad at the ice and our own lack of attention. We see the truck coming and we know this could be bad. But we've got the wheel. We're in control as much as anyone can be.

Not so with our passengers. They're praying and hoping and trusting us to do our best. Sure, if the crash comes, we steer it so we're the one who takes the brunt, but they're still in it.

It's a helpless feeling for that passenger. I know Helen loves me enough that she would do it for me if she could—suffer the knife and the tubes, take the chemo and the nausea, walk daily with the fear. But it's not in her hands. She can only ride along, and pray, and trust me to steer my best.

How I would like to take the fear and uncertainty from her! I can't. When you're the driver, you can't be the passenger, too. I have to trust her, also, to sit quietly and not distract me, to pray hard, to duck when I need to see out her window. I need her to trust me.

It's not totally in my hands. I didn't put the ice there in the dark. I may not be able to control the spin. Maybe that tanker full of fear will hit us yet. But I'm doing my best, and so is she.

Now that I have cancer, I worry about my wife.

. . . I have something to offer.

SOMETHING TO OFFER TO others: my diseased self. I know that there is healing in helping.

I always had myself to offer, of course, and often did. It's my profession, so it wasn't difficult. People expected it of me. That is a problem for ministers, however, and also for their church members. How much is the pastor giving of his or her self because the other person really needs it, and how much is given just because it is required by the job description?

A diseased self is a different self to offer. Only another injured self can see the beauty and holiness in a cancerous self. When it is offered, it is just because we share in the "holeness" of life. We need one another to fill the gaps.

Only a couple of months after my surgery and diagnosis, I wrote a little piece for a national church newspaper. They titled it, "Getting Sick Is Part of Life; Getting Well Is My Ministry." In it I spoke of how I was trying to get well in public, as a sharing of self with my congregation, because my ability to minister to them in conventional ways was going to be limited, at least until my twelve months of chemotherapy were done.

I began to get letters and phone calls from people all over the country in response to that article. Almost all came from other patients or from people who have friends or family members suffering from cancer. A man called from Tulsa, Oklahoma. He told me how he had just about decided to give up, but that my article had given him the strength to go on. Another telephoned from a small town in Iowa. He informed me that he'd had cancer for five years and had told no one; I was the first person he had talked to about it. A woman wrote to tell me of the bravery of her friend as she suffered. I think she just wanted to let someone know of the beauty of that struggle, someone she thought would understand it from the inside. Some wrote to ask for prayers, for themselves or for loved ones. Many fellow patients simply wanted to write a word of encouragement.

I correspond and am in telephone contact with a whole host of new friends. We share good news and bad, comfort and fear, with one another. Although each of us must walk our lonesome valley by ourselves, we do it in the spiritual presence of others who are walking their particular valleys with courage and strength. We are better because we are together. We are together because we share the disease.

I feel that I have been ordained twice. The first time was to the ministry of the church, when Bishop Richard Raines and Rev. Ed Boase and Dr. Otis Collier laid their hands upon me. The second time was to the ministry of cancer, when Drs. Frederic Haynes and Robert Arrol and Alan Hatfield and nurses Kim Wagler and Olivia Parker and Becky Elliott laid their hands upon me.

If you're reading this, it probably means some physician or nurse has laid hands on you and ordained you, also, to this cancer ministry.

Now that I have cancer, there is healing in helping.

. . . *My right leg is bald.*

THAT'S RIGHT, MY LEG! Isn't that a kick? The chemo couldn't get my head, because it's already bald. Most of the men in my family have bald heads and a lot of hair everyplace else. We like it; growing hair is the only way we know to be macho. Now here I am with my hairy chest and my hairy arms and my *one* hairy leg! Thank goodness it's not summer.

I have asked my oncologist and the chemo nurses about it. "Why would the stuff make only my right leg bald?" I inquire.

They have no idea, so they look at me like it's my fault. "Have you been exercising *both* your legs when you take your daily walk?"

I'm a pretty good athlete, but even I can't walk a mile on one leg!

Hair is important to us, isn't it? Most of us dread hair loss more than nausea or mouth sores or the other side effects of chemo. Hair loss shows all the time; the others don't. We make a game of it, or make jokes about it, and wear turbans and wigs and baseball caps. We make the best of it, but we don't like it.

What can you do for a bald leg? Sure, I can keep it covered up, but that's almost unfair. To be really empathetic with my friends in the chemo treatment room, shouldn't I go around in shorts and then wear an ace bandage all up and down my leg? One youngster is bald as a cue ball from his chemo. Last time they were in, his father had shaved his own head, too. They wore matching baseball caps. I liked that. I almost feel guilty when I see someone in a wig. I want to say, "Hey, take a look at my leg. It got me, too," but that would be really weird.

I had hair on my head the first thirty years of my life. It's a shame because it didn't matter much then. Every man in the world in that era, except violinists, wore a crew cut. Crew cuts took almost no work. You went to the barber once a week to get the hedge clippers run over it to keep it flat, and in the morning you ran a hand over it to be sure it was still there. No mirror time necessary.

About thirty, though, I began to go bald. I knew the crew cut would let the bald spot show through like a spotlight. I decided to grow my hair out. I could then comb it over from the side and cover the bald spot. However, I knew that everyone would make fun of me if they noticed this.

So I started growing a beard. In those days, you were considered at least a Communist sympathizer if you had a beard. Everyone I knew was so busy criticizing the hair on the bottom of my head they didn't even notice I was also growing it out on top!

There was one other problem, though. Trimming a beard and growing hair out takes time in front of the mirror. I had never seen so much of myself. It was shocking! I didn't like what I saw.

One day my wife was passing by the bathroom doorway as I worked away on my face in front of the mirror.

"You know," I said, "I really am not very good looking."

"That's right," she replied, and I knew immediately I had made my statement in order to get an entirely different reply from her.

"Hey, wait a minute," I called. "You're my wife. You're not supposed to agree with things like that."

She returned to the door and leaned against the jamb, her arms folded.

"Well, you're never very good looking when you're only looking at yourself," she said, "but you're very handsome when you're looking at me."

She smiled, and I heard the truth in a way I never had before. You're always at your best when you're concentrating on those you love, and who love you, rather than on yourself.

So what am I going to do about this bald leg? I'm going to comb the hair over from the left one to cover it, and I'm not going to let Helen see me do it!

Now that I have cancer, my right leg is bald.

. . . *I've lost my prejudices.*

I WAS NEVER MUCH inclined to prejudge people, at least not along traditional lines of color or religion or nationality. However, I have to admit that I had my reservations about certain other categories of folk: insurance representatives and drug dealers and TV evangelists and telephone solicitors and used car sellers and appliance repairers. I've also been guilty of the most ironic prejudice, the prejudgment of prejudiced people.

When cancer comes, though, how can you hang on to prejudices? Cancer is an equal opportunity disease. It knows no boundaries, not nation or language or race or creed. It strikes a schoolteacher as easily as a mass murderer, a nurse as readily as a hobo, a member of the NAACP as quickly as a knight of the KKK.

One of the best things my mother ever did for me was to insist that each person has to be accepted as an individual, without the cost of the clothes or the color of the skin or the direction of the prayer considered at all. Still, I have had my doubts—about child abusers and hypocrites and falling-down drunks.

Yes, lifestyle makes a difference. So do environmental factors. A smoker is more likely to get lung cancer. A pesticide worker probably takes a higher risk than an accountant. Those aren't the lines over which we usually divide, though, are they? Smokers are both black and white. Pesticide workers are both straight and gay.

One of my friends had to drive thirty miles each week to get her chemotherapy. She is a tall, beautiful woman of great self-composure, at that time in her twenties. Two other women rode with her. One was an elderly, wealthy, patrician lady, a product of the "best" families and schools and beauty salons. The other was a bedraggled, beaten-down woman who looked much older than she was. This unlikely trio went each week to the same hospital for the same treatment, in a VW Beetle yet! As they drove home after their chemo, every few miles one of them would yell "Pit stop." All three would struggle out of the VW to throw up in the ditch along the highway. They took turns holding each other up and passing around the tissues and saying "You look awful," and then laughing like idiots.

I don't think they ever went shopping or dining or to the opera together because of that experience. You don't stop being who you are because you get cancer. More importantly, though, you stop judging who others are.

Isn't it strange, how we divide ourselves one from another, by such superficial categories as the color of our skin and the size of our bank account? Cancer doesn't even look at color or creed or condition. Nor does its treatment. If radiation burns, it will burn the same on Christians and Jews. Chemotherapy nauseates rich and poor alike. Mastectomies leave the chests of black women and white women looking the same.

Now that I have cancer, I just don't have time to judge the lives of others. I'm too busy making sense out of my own. I also know that every other cancer patient is a special sister or brother to me, whether poor or rich, Republican or Democrat, black or white (or red, brown, or yellow), rural or urban, Christian or Jew or secularist. Cancer doesn't have many good faces, but this is one that is almost beautiful. What a relief it is, too. No more energy wasted on judging and prejudging. Just humans together, bound into one cancer-fighting army.

Whoever you are, welcome to the fray.

Now that I have cancer, I can't see your skin or degrees or holy books. All I see is you. You look good, too!

. . . *My attitude is a gift I can give.*

IT'S A GIFT TO those who love me and who care about me. It's perhaps the best gift I can give, because I can't guarantee anything else. I can't say for sure that I'll get cured and stay around here to love them, even though I'm working hard at it. But that's the point, isn't it? I'm doing my best to deal with it, regardless of the outcome.

I'm not sure you have to work at getting cured to give the gift of attitude. A time comes for some when no amount of work will reverse the movement toward the body's death. There is still the gift of attitude, however, in how we look at death and separation.

There is a story of a dying historian, in a day when medicine was primitive and most people died at home. His family had gathered around his bed. His breathing seemed to have stopped. They couldn't find a pulse. They weren't sure whether he was alive or dead. "Feel his feet," someone suggested. "No one ever died with warm feet." From the bed came some muttered last words: "Joan of Arc did." What a gift to his family, what a token of remembrance—of humor, of history, of the kind of man he was.

Another gift we can give is letting others share the process of our getting well. I don't mean necessarily the process of getting cured, because that will not happen for everyone. Not all will be cured, but all can be healed. I'm talking about our relationships, to others and to the world, about forgiveness, about saying good-bye, about taking care of unfinished business, about living in the moment. Allowing our loved ones and friends just to watch us in the process of getting our lives in order is a gift, a way for them to overhear the truth.

Søren Kierkegaard, the Danish philosopher, tells of how he overheard a conversation in a cemetery. He was on the other side of a hedge from a new grave. He made out two voices beside that mound of earth. From the conversation he learned that one voice belonged to a grandfather and the other to his grandson. The man who was son to one and father to the other lay in the grave. The grandfather explained in simple terms about death and new life and memories and healing, terms he would have been embarrassed to use had he known the great and highly recognizable philosopher was listening to him. Kierkegaard said that in those plain words, he overheard the truth, a truth he would not have gotten had he come at it straight on, asking for it, trying to wring it out of his own experience and study.

The truth usually is heard best if it is overheard. Allowing others to overhear, to look over our shoulders as we go about getting well, is a gift we can give now, even if we can give no other.

Our older daughter, Mary Beth, was in her church one Sunday when a man came in during the sermon. He was wild-eyed and carried a case, somewhat like a violin case. He walked down the middle aisle of the long, Gothic-style cathedral, banging the case on the end of each pew as he went. Mary Beth, being a preacher's daughter, always sits up front. In a big church, that means she sits alone; there's enough room for everyone else in the back. So he was even with the second pew, where she sat, before she saw him.

He stopped at the head of the aisle, turned, and looked at everyone with his gleaming eyes. What would he do? Did he have a gun in that case? Would he shoot them all, like madmen do in public places?

The preacher there told me that Mary Beth slipped off her shoes, pulled up her skirt, and got into a low, sprinter's crouch. But then the young man, never revealing what was in the case, walked out again.

I asked Mary Beth about it after I had heard the story from my preacher friend, Paul. "What were you doing?" I said.

"I was getting ready to charge him if he pulled out a gun," she replied.

"Good grief, daughter. You could never have gotten to him before he killed you. You should have hid under the pew."

"Well, I knew that if he had a gun and I charged him, I would die. But I thought that might give Paul and the choir and organist and the others a chance to duck down, to get out the side doors, to run for help. There just wasn't anyone else up there, Daddy. In that place, at that time, I was the one."

When you are the only one, in that place, at that time, you have to take action. In this place, at this time, I'm the only one who can give my loved ones the gift of attitude, the gift of doing my best with what I've got, without denial, to be a healer—for myself and for them.

Now that I have cancer, even though I can't give many gifts, my attitude is a gift I can give.

. . . *I'm a forgiver.*

I'VE ASKED MYSELF, "Why did I get cancer? Have I had some loss that left a vacuum for the disease to fill? Did I need it for some other reason?" The answer surprises me. I got it so I could do some forgiving. Not so I could be forgiven, but so I could be a forgiver, of others and of myself. It is so strange, because I did not know there was anyone I needed to forgive.

I have always been a model child. I spent my entire life before cancer trying to make my parents happy, trying to make them proud of me, trying to take care of them. I didn't even know most of the time that that's what I was doing.

I also don't know why I took that as my unconscious goal in life. It was almost arrogance, deciding I was the parent and they were the children. Except I doubt that a child can truly be arrogant. I was just a little kid, after all, when I started acting that way.

Oh, there were some obvious reasons why I took on that role. We were poor, and I just felt bad my parents and brother and sisters had so little. I even left high school early to work in a factory so I could help with family expenses. I got a lot of praise from the extended family for being "a good boy." In the culture in which I grew up, it was expected the oldest son would act that way.

You see, it was such a "right" thing to do. How could it be wrong? How can it be bad for a boy to work hard and make his parents proud and take care of his family?

I had done that for almost forty years, even while marrying and going to school and raising children and pursuing a career, when I got cancer. Then, suddenly, I could no longer fill any of my old roles with anyone.

About four months after my surgery, when I was well into chemotherapy, my parents had a problem. It was the sort of thing that in the past would have had me on the road in a matter of hours, going a state away to solve it for them, to line up the resources they needed, to take care of them, to be the dutiful son. Now, though, I couldn't. My sisters and brother were many, many states away; they couldn't step in and fill the gap, either. Mother and Dad were left on their own.

The most amazing thing happened: They handled it! They solved the problem. They did what they needed to do, and they did it well.

Wow, did I feel stupid. I'd been messing in their lives all those years, trying to make things better for them, and I was actually making them worse. They didn't need me to take care of them; they needed me to back out so they could take care of themselves. I'd been playing good son, and they'd been playing grateful parents, and neither of us knew it was a bad game.

So, I've forgiven them, and me.

"But wait," you say. (At least I hope you say it; the flow of this will be ruined otherwise, so cooperate.) "Why do you need to forgive them, and yourself, for being in the wrong roles all those years, if neither of you is to blame, if you were just trying to do good? Why not just get on with your lives?"

That I don't know, but the cancer is a clue. I'd been for giving all my life, that was my role. Because it was so deeply buried, so ingrained, I couldn't get out of it. It took cancer to knock me off stride, off balance, out of every normality, to make me realize I couldn't go on that way anymore. I had to stop being for giving and start being forgiving.

I got cancer, you see, so my parents could be set free from their child, and so their child could finally be set free from them. Together, we gave me cancer, in order to cut loose. We didn't have a bad relationship, but we had a wrong relationship. Forgiveness is what puts that which is out of balance into harmony.

Is that really why I got cancer? Isn't it more likely to be fat in my diet, or smoke in the air? I mean, isn't that reaching some? Who knows? What I do know is that the presence of cancer caused a very important thing to happen, for me and for my parents. In that sense, that's why I got cancer, so I could be a forgiver.

I don't expect you to have a similar story to tell at all, but I suspect that cancer is giving you a chance to become a forgiver. Look deep. See what patterns and relationships of your life are no longer possible because of the cancer. Then forgive.

Now that I have cancer, I'm a forgiver.

. . . I understand about "big guys."

IN THOSE LAST WEEKS, Benny always called me "Big Guy" or "The Tall One." I knew he wasn't making fun of me, but it was still hard to understand. Yes, I am a big guy. Six feet and one inch, when I had all my hair. Too many pounds to be called slender anymore. I'm the kind of guy you put at first base when he gets too slow to play anywhere else.

Ben himself, though, was truly a big guy. His curly, steel-gray hair topped out more than six inches above my neater hairline. He weighed about two hundred and eighty, and not much of it was fat. In high school football he was all-state. When I hugged him I feared my nose would get a belly button bruise. He was a giant, so why did he call *me* "Big Guy"?

He was a few years older, but we got sick about the same time. His was his heart; mine was cancer. He was given six months. They told me a year or two.

He accepted his diagnosis but not mine. So we entered into an unspoken pact. I would get well for both of us. He would die for both of us.

Through my year of treatment he knew my chemotherapy schedule better than I did. He never failed to telephone during my week of nausea or my week of mouth sores. His statement was always, "I just want you to get well."

He defied the odds and confounded the physicians, as he always did. He lived fifteen months, not six, enough to see me through the chemotherapy and to hear the oncologist say that, at least for now, I was "clean." Then he timed his death so I could attend his funeral the day before I left for my "end of chemo" celebration trip.

It was in the last six weeks of our pact that he started

calling me "Big Guy" or "The Tall One." My chemotherapy was complete, and I could visit him in the cardiac hospice each day. One or the other of his grown sons would always be there, each one taller than I. Strangely, the shortest man in the room was the "Big Guy."

Benny and I always acted in a way that befitted big guys, when others were around. We were a macho pair, swaggering down the hospital halls together, impressing the nurses with our deep voices and amazingly funny stories, talking masculine stuff, like pickup trucks and oil viscosity. When we were alone, however, we talked about our wives and children and whether our grandchildren would remember us. When we were alone, we held hands. When we were alone, we prayed. When we were alone, we cried. I didn't feel that big.

It was then that I understood. It really *is* lonely at the top, up where yours is the only head because you're the biggest guy around. It's hard, always being the biggest. People expect you to *act* head and shoulders above the rest, not just stand that way.

Remember the curse they put on Jesus? "He does all things well" (Mark 7:37). How could anyone live up to an expectation like that? No wonder he got into so much trouble. I remember when I was "a promising young man." It was frightening. No one tells you what the promises are, but everyone expects you to keep them. How much worse to have it said of you, "He does all things well."

Maybe that's why Jesus called Peter "Big Guy." (The more common translation is "rock.") Peter was smaller than Jesus in every way that counted. Some people even think it was a slightly cruel joke, calling Peter "Big Guy." When accusations came in the night, he didn't have the heart of a mouse. Jesus knew what he was getting, though. He had no illusions about Peter. Jesus just needed someone to remind him that he wasn't alone at the top.

Jesus had a pact with Peter, too, just as Benny had with me. Peter would do the getting well, the getting healed, for both, and Jesus would do the dying for both.

People think that big guys (and big gals) get through life without pain or problem, whether the size is physical or financial or spiritual. It's not true. Even the largest of the large, the strongest of the strong, has to have someone else to call "Big Guy." You need someone you can look up to, even if you have to kneel to do it.

Now that I have cancer, I understand about "Big Guys."

12. WHEN IT'S TIME TO LOOK INSIDE

(DEALING WITH OUR FEELINGS)

Now that I have cancer . . .

. . . *I can't decide what to buy.*

IS BUYING A NEW book an act of faith or an act of stupidity? Can I get enough good out of a new shirt, or should I just try to wear out the old ones while I can? What about that World War II leather pilot's jacket I've wanted since I was eight years old? I found a great one, just like the originals, and it's "only" $250, the lowest price I've seen.

How in the world, though, can I justify a new shirt or a pilot's jacket if I die before I get much wear out of it? Nobody else in the family wears my size. They'd just be more things for my wife to get rid of. Besides, do I have a right to spend anything at all on myself when so much money is going into my treatments?

Health care costs a bundle. Doctors and hospitals are mostly covered because we have good insurance. There are all kinds of extra costs, however, that go with illness: telephone, special food, mileage and motels and restaurants for out-of-town hospital trips. My salary continues, but who knows about the future?

I'm sick from cancer, and I'm also sick of being practical. I want to buy that book just because I want to read it. I want that shirt because I'm tired of looking at all my old ones. That pilot's jacket means more to me than just keeping warm on a winter day. I want to think I'm special enough to be worth a new shirt or a new book.

How do I make these decisions? How do I make any decisions at all?

This is going to sound simplistic, but we make our decisions through love. The good decisions are love in action. The bad ones are love gone wrong. All our decisions, even the bad ones, are made through love. Love is why we have decisions to make at all.

Think of cancer in that light. Cancer is just growth gone wrong. There's nothing wrong with growth. We automatically think of it as good. There's so much of growth that is right and necessary. We cannot live without growth. When it starts coloring outside the lines, however, when the cells start dividing like they're trying to fight off snakes, tumors result.

A bad decision is love gone wrong. Love makes us want to be in a relationship with what is loved, makes us hug and hold and admire. Love also makes us hurt when we can't have what we love, when we can't skip like lambs upon the hills with whatever or whoever makes us joyous.

Growth gone wrong is disease. Love gone wrong is disease. Love gone wrong makes bad decisions, choices that hurt instead of heal.

Cancer decisions are love decisions. Like any other love decision, we may make it poorly. We might make it to protect ourselves from the pain of loss or the agony of closeness rather than making it to increase joy. Either way, it's a decision because of love.

It's funny how cancer affects love decisions. Some are so clear you can see your face in them. Others are like looking into a puddle where someone's stirred up all the mud with a stick.

The big decisions are the easy ones, aren't they? Do I want to get well? Do I want to live in wholeness? Do I want to be part of the solution instead of part of the problem?

The little decisions, like what to buy—how can we tell what's a loving choice? I don't know. I do know, however, that each decision is a love decision and that each of us is loved, including me.

Now that I have cancer, I can't decide what to buy,
but I know that love is a gift.

. . . I have to remember that I'm not a disease.

TOO MANY PEOPLE FORGET THAT.

"I may have cancer, but cancer doesn't have me." When I was in the hospital, recovering from my surgery, I knew I had it made when my wife reported a conversation she overheard at the nurses' desk. They were saying, "The gall bladder in 604 needs some juice, and the amputation in 612 is complaining again, but the congestion case in 630 is beginning to settle down. And, oh, Mr. McFarland is ready for bed, too."

I wasn't just a disease; I was a person! I had a name!

If I am not just a disease, then I am not identified by the disease. Cancer is not my middle, or even first, name. That means that a cure for the disease is not the first priority. The most important thing for my life is healing.

If I am cured of cancer but try to live an unwholesome life, I am not healed, and so I am not me. I am still identified by the disease, either by having it or not having it. Jesus once said, "What does it profit you to gain the whole world if you forfeit your soul?" What value is there in cure if it only leads to a longer meaningless life?

That doesn't mean I ignore or deny the cancer. It's as much a part of me as being male, white, and a Reds fan. I'll always have the fear and challenge of cancer. But that fear and challenge can be what leads to healing.

By healing I mean getting life right, being in a right relationship with God and the others in your universe and your own true self. In Larry LaShan's words, you "sing your own song." If that wholeness is there, every moment seems like a sudden eternity rather than a past to regret and a future to fret. Maybe that is what religious folks mean when they talk about eternal life.

I sometimes say that I have lived more in the few months I've had cancer than I did in all my previous years. That doesn't mean the former years were not good. There was some wonderful loving that went on in those years. But the intensity of healing, in the face of death, has been a great gift. I thank God for my cancer.

Some people, hearing that, will undoubtedly say, "Now that you have cancer, you're crazy!" But some of you will understand: Now that I have cancer, I am not just a disease, and I am not identified by it. It is just the occasion of learning my real identity.

Now that I have cancer, I'm not a disease.

. . . *I want to forget about cancer*.

IT'S EVERYWHERE. I stand in the grocery checkout line, scanning the tabloids. "Miracle Cancer Cure Fails Siamese Twin Mother from Mars." "Brown Rice Causes Cancer," according to "noted Chinese healer Toe Foo." I get home and fetch the regular newspaper out of the bushes. The front page of the "Living" section is dedicated to "Ten Anti-Cancer Recipes Using Brown Rice." The *Perriwinkle People* cartoon strip features a hairless dog on chemo.

On the way home I pass the Déjà View Theater. The marquee proclaims "Cancer Ward Nurses from Hell" and "Losing It All," the touching, romantic story of an oncologist and her older but wealthy patient. Four letters, all addressed to me but each with a different and exotic spelling of my name, tell me I can "lick" cancer in my lifetime if I just make a donation to the Meredith Lovely Cancer Research Foundation. (How does Ms. Lovely, famous actress and accessories activist, know how long my lifetime is, anyway?) *Backward Trails* magazine tells of "Thirty-Three Bed and Breakfast Vacations You Can Take to Avoid Cancer."

I switch on the TV and see a public service announcement from the Nuclear Energy Regulating Down South (NERDS) Agency titled "Carcinogens Can Be Good for You." I give that up and try public radio, where a woman from the Tobacco Research Institute for Profits Entirely (TRIPE) is telling three lung cancer patients that there's no real evidence her product had anything to do with it, and besides, taking risks is the American way, and who are they to deny others a chance at the same experience, anyway?

Someone I met eleven years ago at a party for the neighbor's schnauzer telephones to tell me his Aunt Sonya had cancer and lived a surprisingly long time, although he can't remember if it was weeks or years. I riffle through the mail and find that my book club is featuring the latest by I. M. Wilde, M.D., titled *Schemo Your Way Through Chemo with My New Product, "Dreamo."*

I guess all this stuff about cancer was in the air before I got it, but I can't remember it. Oh, sure, the occasional odd article, a guest once in a while on the Fill with Okra show, but all the time?

"I've got cancer, but cancer doesn't have me." I don't want every picture of my life bordered in black, every line in my story penned by chemo, every note in my song sung by radiation.

I'm a cancer patient, sure, but I'm more than a victim. I'm a real human being, with hopes and fears that have nothing to do with cancer. I worry about my children, the ozone, the economy, whether I can make the car payment. They are the same worries I had B.C., before cancer. I rejoice in a joke, a well-turned phrase, the face of an old friend, a snatch of a "golden oldie" on the radio, the touch of my wife's lips. They are the same joys I had B.C.

I can't forget about cancer entirely, and I don't want to. That would not be healthy. Cancer is part of my life. But it's only my body that has cancer all the time. It's okay for my spirit to be free from it once in a while. Yours, too.

Now that I have cancer, I want to forget about cancer.

. . . *I'm a person.*

NOT JUST A PATIENT.

It's hard to know what to call us, isn't it? Are we victims? Patients? Respondents? Conquerors?

Yes, we're victims. We've been attacked. Bad things are happening to us. Sometimes we certainly feel victimized. But if victim is all we are, then there's no hope for us.

We're patients while we're being treated, but we're not just patients, and sometimes we're not very patient at all! We're not patients all the time; certainly we hope to be past treatment someday.

Bernie Siegel suggests "cancer respondent." That's not bad, but it's not very clear. It doesn't roll off the tongue easily, either.

Conqueror? Well, yes, some of us, at least some of the time, but that's not a word that can be used about us automatically, just because we have cancer. Besides, the apostle Paul reminds us that the important thing is to be *more* than conquerors (Romans 8:37).

I prefer to think of myself simply as a person, like every other person, except I happen to have cancer. I'm a cancer person.

Now I know that's not a very good solution to the name problem either. It's certainly not going to catch on and sweep the nation. It has its drawbacks, just like the other names. Perhaps we're not supposed to be able to find an adequate name, and perhaps that is the point!

When Moses asked God to tell him a name, one he could take back to the people to convince them he really had met up with the divine and that the commandments had come from God, not just from Moses' own brain, God refused.

"I am who I am," God said. "Tell them that."

God didn't want to be tied down to a single name; that was too limiting.

Names are important. They can hurt or they can heal. That's why minority groups and others marginal to power are especially concerned about what name they are known by, because they are particularly vulnerable to being dismissed through some uncomplimentary name.

My family name is Scots-Irish. When the Irish first immigrated to America, they were very poor, and uncultured and uneducated. Because most of the Irish family names began with "Mc," we were dismissed as "micks," as in, "He's only a mick." Saloonkeepers and shopkeepers put signs in their windows saying "No dogs or micks allowed." Help-wanted signs often bore the legend, "No Irish need apply." We weren't people, we were just a name.

An experiment was done with grade school teachers. They were asked to grade essays. Some of the papers bore unusual student names associated with minority groups. Others had standard American childhood names, such as Bobby and Susie. Although they were the same essays, "Bobby" and "Susie" got much better grades than the "irregular" names. The teachers reacted to the names and the qualities they associated with them, not just to the essays.

"I am who I am." Perhaps that's a good enough name for any of us. Descriptive names have some value; it would be difficult to converse without them. Personal names have value, too. They are shorthand versions of our own stories. When I hear "Babe Ruth" or "Abraham Lincoln" or "Elizabeth Taylor," I immediately know the story, the lifeline, to which that name refers. Category names, though, tend to hide our individual narratives, obscure who we are in our glorious uniqueness.

Now that I have cancer, I'm a person, not just a patient.

. . . I don't get mad when I forget to switch the magnets on the dishwasher.

WELL, NOT AS MUCH, ANYWAY.

There's nothing quite as maddening as getting halfway through unloading the dishwasher only to find that the dishes are dirty. I've put four plates, six glasses, five cups, and eight bowls into the cupboards, and they were dirty!

"I'm innocent," I scream at the dishwasher police. "The clean magnet was on the front. How was I to know?"

Yes, I know I should be able to tell by looking, but my wife rinses everything until it's almost clean before it goes in the dishwasher. So, it's switch the magnet to "dirty" and take everything out of the cupboard and put it back in the dishwasher.

We have two magnets. One is brown and has a picture of a sloppy duck and proclaims "Dirty." The other is green and shows a nice, polite swan. It says "Clean" right across the top. It's simple to keep them properly organized. Just take the "clean" magnet off the front of the machine and stick it onto the side when the last clean dish has been put away. Then take the "dirty" magnet off the side of the machine and move it to the front. Simple, right?

Wrong! For some reason, no one else in the family remembers to do this. I alone take on this arduous task of remembrance and action. I am the best magnet switcher in the family, perhaps in the entire county. I never forget!

Except sometimes—and there's the problem. It's just awfully hard to be perfect. At anything. I have my whole identity invested in switching those magnets at the proper times, however.

Those magnets say a great deal about who I am. I am an organized person. I am efficient. I get the most out of my time. I'm busy, so I must be important. The world would have a most difficult time getting along without me. How would the world's magnets get switched otherwise?

I heard a friend ask a whole group of people what had been their most successful day of work ever. They named days on which they had accomplished great things: got married, turned out 347 parts on the assembly line, flunked an entire class of students, plowed eighty acres, made five thousand dollars. Then he asked, "What was Jesus' most successful day of work, the day he fed five thousand people or the day he was crucified?"

You don't have to be a Christian believer to understand that, do you? Those five thousand people went full for one day. But Jesus' crucifixion brought into being a two-thousand-year church. Sometimes that looks like a better day of work than it does on others, but you have to admit that Jesus' failure that day, his loss, was powerfully successful.

Being perfect, being successful, even being efficient, isn't all it's cracked up to be. You can get a whole lot done, even be sure the magnets are switched every time, and not have accomplished very much. Maybe the successful day is the one where we just get by: survive the chemo or radiation, show a little kindness to ourselves and those around us, grow a little toward wholeness, live in the present moment, which is the eternal now. Perhaps it doesn't matter that much if the magnets don't get switched, if perfection is not achieved.

I suspect the dishes will forgive me. I know God will.

Perhaps I'll even forgive myself, if I have any time left over for it after I get this magnet thing straightened out.

Now that I have cancer, I've learned to go a little easier on perfection. I don't get mad when I forget to switch the magnets—well, not as much, anyway.

13. WHEN YOU WONDER WHAT IT MEANS

(LOOKING FOR ANSWERS)

Now that I have cancer . . .

. . . I'm at war against myself.

I AM A SCARRED and scorched battlefield. I am also both of the armies that charge from foxhole to trench and back again across that weary field of battle. I am the body that has cancer, and I am the cancer that lives in the body. The cancer is a part of me that has run amok, but it is still a part of me, for all that. In trying to destroy the cancer cells, I am also attempting to destroy a part of me. Some of me has to die if the rest of me is to live. The only way I can be more whole is if I am less whole.

No wonder cancer is the most confusing disease! Cancer is also, I think, the most spiritual of diseases.

Life in the spirit is a constant letting go in order to take hold, a continual giving up in order to take in. The spirit is just like a hand. If it is balled up into a fist, holding tight to what it has, all it is useful for is hitting and hurting. However, if it is open, whatever it holds is free to go, but also it is ready to receive whatever might be given.

There is a physical part of me, the cancer, that must be killed, cut out, eradicated, that my body might live. So also there is a spiritual part of me that has to be destroyed for my own health and wholeness. Just as with the body, my spirit will be more whole if I am less whole.

This is the great lesson of cancer, the spiritual disease. I'm not just at war with myself in my body; I'm at war with myself in the spirit, too.

I'm not saying there is no "devil," no force of evil that exists outside us. There seems to be pretty good evidence that evil has a life of its own, invading and intruding where it truly is not wanted.

There is evil *within* us as well, however, that which would kill the soul as well as the body. Christians have traditionally called this "original sin." H. L. Mencken, the great American cynic, used to say that original sin was the only Christian doctrine for which there is empirical evidence. I think he was wrong about it being the only one, but he was certainly right about the evidence for it!

We don't *want* to be battlefields. Of course not! People are not meant to live constantly with tension and confusion. We want to be able to choose sides and cheer for one team or the other.

Mayor La Guardia of New York founded the famed City Center of Theater and Drama. Someone once asked him why, because he had worked so hard to create the center, he never went to the ballet there. He said, "I'm a guy who likes to keep score. With the ballet, I never know who's ahead." Yes! We like to keep score. Cancer is more like ballet than basketball, however. If we have to shoot at both baskets, how can we know if we're winning?

Somehow we have to deal with this contradiction. If we don't acknowledge the inward battle and enter into it, if we try for a separate peace, then we can't get well. We can choose one side or the other and resolve the tension, but we give up a part of our own story when we do.

There's an old tale about a hermit in the mountains who was supposed to be exceptionally wise. Some of the local boys decided to put him to the test. One of them held a small, live bird in his closed hand, then asked the old man if it were alive or dead. If he said it was alive, the boy would crush the bird in his fist and show it as dead. If the hermit said it was dead, he would open his hand and let it fly free. Either way they would confound the wise man and prove him stupid. But when they put the question to him, the old man simply replied, "It is as you will."

Am I the cancer or the cancer fighter? I am both. Strange and contradictory as it is, that is my story. It is not something outside myself but a part of me that I must let go in order to live, not just to be cured in the body but to be healed in myself. I accept the battle and know that its outcome is as I will.

Now that I have cancer, I am at war against myself.
I trust that I shall win.

. . . *I live in the present.*

ROSE MARY SHEPHERD, MY cancer shepherd, was in our bathroom. She noticed a book I had left there on my "morning misery" table. Its subtitle is *Getting Back to Normal When You Have Cancer.* She snorted as she returned to the living room. "There's no such thing as getting back to normal when you have cancer," she said. "Things are changed forever."

I know what she means. I agree with her. Mostly, I don't want to get back to normal, if normal is the careless way I went through life before cancer. I just took so much for granted. I didn't really enjoy most of my life, even though the ingredients for joy were certainly there.

Don't get me wrong; my life fit me well. It wasn't like a shirt that chafes around the collar. But it was like a checklist on a clipboard: I did something and checked it off and went on to the next thing on the list. College? Check. Marriage? Check. Children? Check. Career? Check. I was focused mostly on the future, on what was coming up next on the list, instead of really experiencing what was happening to me right then.

Senator Green of Rhode Island held a seat in Congress up into his nineties. One night he was at a party when his hostess caught him peering into his date book. "Now, Senator Green," she admonished, "are you already thinking about where you're going next?" "No," he replied, "I'm trying to find out where I am now." Not a bad idea.

Bible scholar Günther Bornkamm notes that in Jesus' time, all his people were focused either on the past or on the future. There were those, like the Pharisees, who tried so hard to live by the law they had inherited from generations past that they failed to get into the now. Then there were those who looked forward so eagerly to the apocalypse, when God would bring an end to the world and separate the righteous from the unrighteous, that they also failed to live in the now. Jesus' accomplishment, Bornkamm says, was that he made it possible for people to live in the present without denying the reality and importance of either the past or the future.

I think God used my cancer in that way, freeing me from fretting the future (worrying about what I'm supposed to do next) and regretting the past (worrying about things I left undone) so that I can live right now. I get more "right now" time in a day than I used to get in a year.

I think that surely this is what is meant by eternal life, not just that life goes on forever and ever, but the quality in which all the future and all the past come together in the present, when all of life is right here, in the eternal now.

When I was young and working with college students only a few years younger than I, I invited one of my personal heroes, Richard Campbell Raines, to lead a weekend retreat for the students. He did so, but with reluctance. He was seventy at the time and had just retired. He said, "I'm not sure I can relate to the students. I live in the present age, but the present age doesn't live in me."

He was probably the best present I ever gave those students. They were delighted that at seventy he had just learned to water-ski, something he'd always wanted to do and never had time for until he retired. He and his age were present to the students in that weekend, and they loved him for it.

I think I understand, especially now that I am older, what he meant. I sometimes feel alien in this world. My internal gyroscope was crafted in an age when horses pulled plows and it was a big thing to have a radio and men went off to fight a war of righteousness in Europe and Asia. The present age does not live in me.

I do live in the present, though, just as Richard Raines did every day of his life. I think that's why he was a hero to me. His present and his presence were so full because he packed all of his vitality and experience into each moment he lived. We don't have to live in the present age to live in the present moment.

The present. Think of its two meanings together. It is both a gift and the now. There's no other time that you can receive a present except in the present, and the only present that can give true joy is the present. The present is a present from God.

Now that I have cancer, I am freed to live in that eternal now, the present.

. . . *I have hope.*

I SUPPOSE IT IS possible to have hope without a chronic illness or some similar disaster, but I don't think I ever did it before. I had a lot of wishes, but hope didn't even occur to me as something I needed.

The apostle Paul, in his letter to the Romans (5:3–5), says that hope comes as the result of suffering. Not directly, of course. Paul says suffering produces endurance, and endurance produces character, and character produces hope. So suffering is strained through endurance and character, kind of like carrots through a colander, to produce hope.

Frankly, I'm not sure about endurance and character in my case. It seems to me those need to be chosen to be real. I suspect whatever endurance and character I have developed as a result of my cancer aren't legitimate. They are there because I have no choice. There are plenty of days I'd gladly give up the cancer and go back to being a spineless nonendurer and a weak-kneed character. I endure, and show more character than I really want to, simply because I have to.

Hope is different, however. If I had to choose between cancer with hope and no cancer but no hope, I'd take the cancer in order to keep the hope. I don't want to disagree with so eminent an authority as Paul, but I think we can have hope even if there are considerable suspicions about our endurance and our character.

It's extremely difficult to define what I mean by hope. I've cast about looking for the right words, but I find hope is more real as a feeling than as a mental concept. The best I can do is this: Hope is the affirmation of life, not just as a fact of existence in this body and in this world but as a reality that transcends the barriers that our skins and the ozone layer set up. Hope is saying "yes" to the whole of life, even if we can see only parts of it. If life is real, then it is real regardless of the container it's kept in.

It's hard for us to see beyond our present containers—our bodies and our world and our years—because they are all we know. Certainly we cannot prove there is anything else. But hope says life is so real and so important that these temporary limits can't be the final word. Hope doesn't need proof in order to know. Hope, like faith, "had its reasons that reason does not know."

I think what distinguishes hope from wishing is that the real object of hope is wholeness: wholeness in relationship to our own true selves, to other people, to the world around us, and, yes, to God. Indeed, wholeness can be described as simply being in the presence of God, although we might use different words for God. Wishing is wanting, longing for something to be different, to look out into the yard and see a pony where there was only a bare spot before. Hoping is trusting that the bare spots will be filled, because the one who is in all and through all will see us through it all. Our hope is in the one who knows what we need, regardless of what we wish for.

Perhaps a story will explain this better than theories. Stories usually do.

William and Mary College, in Virginia, was damaged and closed during the Civil War. After the war it opened but was closed again for seven years. Despite the fact that there were no students or faculty and that the buildings had fallen into disrepair, the president every morning went out to ring the bell. That's hope.

Now that I have cancer, I have hope.

14. WHEN IT'S TIME TO MOVE TOWARD HEALING

(HITTING STRIDE)

Now that I have cancer . . .

. . . I cry a lot.

I'VE NEVER BEEN MUCH of a weeper. I've certainly felt like letting the tears flow once in a while, but I learned early that tears were not acceptable. Even in the darkness of a theater, when the hero's head disappeared in murky water and only his white hat floated slowly toward the shore, even then I squeezed tight upon my popcorn and my eyelids and told the tears to stay put.

I must have been about seven or eight when I saw *Lassie,* the original film version. I can still remember Lassie leaving bloody footprints on the rocks. I wanted so much to cry openly, to share that noble dog's pain. I didn't, though. I clenched my fists and my eyes and I kept all my sorrow inside. I've wanted to cry for Lassie ever since. Only now, as I write these words, am I able to do so.

I envy women when it comes to crying. My wife and my daughters are good criers. If some scene or action or word reaches in and shakes their hearts, you know it by the streams on their cheeks. They might not believe this, but I've never doubted that tears are good. They know I'm uncomfortable with crying, so they try not to overdo it in my presence. I've always known they cried behind my back, though, and I've always wished I could slip in a few tears behind my back, too.

Now that I have cancer, it seems like I have permission to cry. Oh, I still prefer not to do it in public. I'm not sure folks would understand. They might think I lost my marbles or stepped on a tack. I'm talking about permission to myself, permission to cry when I feel like it.

Sure, some of my weeping is because of anesthesia hangover. Maybe chemotherapy has a tear side effect, even. I am sure, however, that I weep now because everything is so beautiful.

I walk my dog down beside St. John's church, the one that looks like it belongs in a German village. I peer up at its tower and stained glass, through my chemo-stuck eyelids, and I cry. I see a finch at the thistle feeder or a squirrel scampering up the TV antenna, and I cry. I examine the face of my wife or see a friend coming toward me or watch Ken Griffey Jr. run down a sure hit and throw the runner out, and I cry.

When I cry, it seems like everything is in balance, in right relationship with all other things, that I'm right at the heart of love. So much is wondrously beautiful, I can't even begin to tell about it. No words are adequate. So I have to cry.

I know there are tears of sadness and bitterness and grief, but I'm not sure they are very different from the tears of beauty. We cry only because of love—because of its absence or its presence. In that way, tears are the sure sign of the reality of love.

I came home one evening when our daughters were teenagers to find them rocking back and forth on the living room sofa, arms locked around each other, weeping as if their hearts were truly broken. Gently I tried to get my arms around them and whispered, "What's wrong? Why are you crying?"

Katie looked at me over Mary Beth's shoulder, with streaming eyes, and choked out, "I don't know. She hasn't told me yet."

We don't really have to know why another is crying in order to share the love and beauty, do we? Tears unite us in the ways of love and take us into the depth of beauty.

Now that I have cancer, I cry a lot—and when I cry,
I know everything is okay.

. . . *I say good-bye.*

I DROVE THROUGH HOOPESTON, Illinois, where we once lived, and I realized I might never see those tree-lined streets again. They hold good memories for me. Our daughters were teenagers there; they learned to drive on those streets. Our older daughter, Mary Beth, graduated from the big, yellow-brick high school there. We loved walking down those streets on a Friday after supper, the four of us under a canopy of old and sheltering trees, to the welcoming little library, where we would check out our weekend books. The people who live in the houses that line those flat, prairie streets were very kind to us, especially during the several months when Helen's mother was dying.

As I drove over the massaging bricks and attention-grabbing potholes, I understood that I might never be in Hoopeston again, except in my mind. I needed to say good-bye to those streets, although not to their memories.

So I said, "Good-bye, Hoopeston. I'm glad you were a part of my life, and I thank you for those good years you gave us. I may see you again, perhaps many times, who knows? But if I don't, that's okay. I hold you in my heart. Please remember me in yours."

Helen and I walked together on the winding paths of the Indiana University campus in Bloomington. IU is where we met and married. We made friends there who remain close and dear to us. I recall those gentle hills and limestone buildings with great affection. Dogwood and redbud trees in bloom always make me want to study for exams. My college years opened to me doors of scholarship and friendship and love that I did not even know existed.

As we left, I said, "Good-bye, IU. I love you still, but I know I may never see you again. I hope that's not true, because I would like to return to this wonderful well to slake my thirst many times. But if I don't, if this is the last time for us to be together, that's okay."

I'm not quite sure why I need to say these tentative farewells to the places of my past. I'm not even sure I need to be there in person to wave that fond good-bye. Perhaps doing it in my mind would be enough.

I do know that commitment to life as unfinished business is one of the marks of a long-term survivor. Saying these interim farewells is, I think, a piece of unfinished business.

When I was told I would be dead "in a year or two," my first thought was, "I can't even use up my return address labels in a year or two." Think of that: They are not useful to anyone but me, and to me only if I'm alive. I figured one of my main tasks of unfinished business would be to use up those labels. The problem is that every organization in the world that wants money from me, and there is no organization in the world that doesn't, keeps sending me more return address labels as a little gift to try to shame me into shelling out some bucks. My unfinished business will take two hundred years at this rate.

Occasionally someone says, "What do you think the best age for a child is? Infant? Three? Wouldn't you like to have them cute like that again for just a day?" We always say, "No, the age they are right now is the best age, because it's the one they're supposed to be."

Life is always a process of letting go of what has been so we can take hold of what will be. That doesn't mean we forget the past. Even old folks whose minds have left them keep in their bones and tissues the remembrance of all the places they have been. We cannot live in the past, however. God is always moving us forward.

Cancer is a forceful reminder of that truth, and I am thankful for the reminder. So I say my tentative farewells. Each one reminds me that I live in an in-between time. In-between is not a bad place to be.

Now that I have cancer, I say good-bye.

. . . I'm a captive of the morning.

IN MY OWN BATHROOM.

One-third of my colon is gone. That means my bowels move three to five times every morning, in the first three to four hours after the dog has gotten me up to let her out for the same reason. (I know I talk about this a lot. I know I've written about it elsewhere. That's because it has become the center post around which my schedule revolves.) That in itself is not so bad. The real problem is that I get only thirty to ninety seconds' notice when it happens.

Think about what that means for planning a day. I can't be more than thirty seconds from a bathroom, so I have to stay at home until I'm certain my semicolon is acceptable in public. Sure, there are restrooms other places, but it takes more than sixty seconds to get to them, and what if there's a line? I can't find a car company that's willing to replace the driver's seat with a toilet, not even the Japanese. (Apparently their knack for innovation goes only so far.) So, if I need to leave the house at 8:30, I have to get up by 5:30, preferably 4:30.

I can't go to breakfast meetings anymore. In fact, I can't go out to breakfast. We can't spend the night with friends or family unless they have a bathroom that's available to me alone. Before cancer, if I had a 9 A.M. meeting a couple of hours away, I just got up at 6, had some breakfast, and drove. Now I have to travel the night before, stay at a motel, and have some breakfast with me that I can eat when I get up at 5. Needless to say, I have to choose very carefully which meetings and events I attend, because of both time and expense.

Some cancer patients face much greater changes in their routines. For others, the outward alterations are few. All of us are changed, however. Even if we peer into the mirror and see the same body we had before cancer. Even if we look at our appointment books and find no differences in our daily comings and goings. Nonetheless, we *are* changed. We are reminded of the changes in varying ways, but changes there are. We are aliens, a different race, from the planet Cancer. We look like everyone else, but we are not.

Some try to deny the change, to act as though all is "normal," whatever that might be, as though nothing even happened. "Cancer? What cancer?" Others let the changes take over, organizing their lives around cancer and its demands. They see themselves only as victims. Either way, cancer is the dominator, the center, the only reality we acknowledge, whether it is hidden or all too obvious.

My colon is a constant reminder that I am a changed person. Cancer has made my life different, forever. I try to make that work for me instead of against me. It is clear that there are things I cannot do now, at least at certain times, that I was able to do before. But what new things can I do now that my life is different? How can I use that morning time in ways to enhance life rather than just by complaining about the changes?

The only sure reality in this life is change. We can ride its wave and see where it takes us, or we can be dragged screaming along with it, but change there will be. Our particular changes are caused by cancer, but cancer is not our cause. Love is found in the rapids, among the rocks, as surely as in the quiet pools. And sometimes there, it is much more exhilarating!

Jacob wrestled with the angel and ended up with a permanent limp, but he got a blessing from that encounter. The limp was a reminder of the blessing. Every step he took, Jacob knew he wasn't a "normal" man. You can't wrestle with an angel, even the angel of death, without knowing you have been changed forever.

Jacob had his limp. I have my semicolon. Some have a lopsided bosom or a lonely kidney. For some the mark on the body is gone completely, but the shape of the angel remains on the soul.

I may never have cancer again, but I'll never be free of it. It's my companion forever. There will always be the worry, and there will always be the blessing.

Now that I have cancer, I am a captive of the morning. It's morning when the day begins.

. . . *I want to pretend that everything is still the same.*

I'M RECOVERING FROM AN operation, that's all. Nothing is different. I don't need to prioritize my time, or conserve my strength, or meditate, or read wellness books, or go to support group. Everything is going to go back to the way it was. The more I act "natural," the sooner my life will be back to normal, I tell myself.

I know it's not true, though. Life will never be the same for me again. I might live a normal life span, whatever that is, but I'll still have to take the tests and watch for the symptoms.

Being a cancer person is like being an alcoholic. Even if you've been dry for five years, or ten or twenty, you're still an alcoholic. You can't take that first drink, regardless of how small. You start every meeting by saying, "I'm an alcoholic."

We might get past the stage of being a cancer patient, being treated, perhaps even being tested, but I suspect we never stop being a cancer person. There's always a piece of the mind that remembers and wonders.

More importantly, we are changed by the experience, whether we want to be or not, and probably even if we can't tell the difference.

One piece of conventional wisdom observes that as we grow older we become more like ourselves. Cancer is an interruption of that process of becoming more like ourselves, an opportunity to go in some other direction if we wish. What happens in our bodies with the onset of cancer may be out of our control, but what happens in our hearts is not.

So even though I want to act like nothing has changed, it has. Now I'm faced with deciding what the change will be. Will I become more open, more spiritual, more loving? Or will I be a denier, and let my denial eat at my spirit the same way the cancer has eaten at my body—secret, steady, eroding.

I once heard someone say that life is far too much trouble unless you can live it for something big. I would add that cancer is far too much trouble unless you can use it for a change in the direction you need to go.

Maybe it's a change you've always wanted to make and just never had the energy or the courage. Perhaps it's a change that is only now occurring as a possibility. It may even be a change that is forced upon you by the circumstances. Whatever, it's your cancer, so it's your change.

I heard about a frog who was hopping down a dirt road. There were two long ruts in the road, worn there by big trucks that occasionally had to use the road. As he hopped along, he spied a friend sitting down at the bottom of one of the ruts.

"What are you doing down there?" he asked. "That could be dangerous."

"Yes, I know," sighed his friend, "but I fell in here by accident, and I've tried and tried to jump out, but I'm just too tired. It is impossible for me to get out."

The first frog went down to the pond to get some help, only to see his little frog friend arriving minutes later. What a surprise.

"What happened?" he asked. "I thought you weren't able to get out of that rut by yourself?"

"Well," replied his friend, "a truck came along in that rut, and I *had* to get out."

Now that I have cancer, I want to pretend that everything is the same, but it's not. That is, at least potentially, cancer's gift, to get me out of my rut.

. . . *I believe in miracles.*

LEE ATWATER WAS A mean guitarist and a mean campaign manager for the first George Bush. He believed in destroying the political opposition in any way possible—not just in beating them but in obliterating them. He took great pride in being nasty. He was only forty when he died of a malignant brain tumor. Before his death, he wrote these words:

> I acquired more wealth, power, and prestige than
> most. But you can acquire all you want and still
> feel empty. . . . It took a deadly illness to put me
> eye to eye with that truth, but it is a truth that
> the country, caught up in its ruthless ambitions
> and moral decay, can learn on my dime. I don't
> know who will lead us through the nineties, but
> they must be made to speak to this spiritual
> vacuum at the heart of American society, this
> tumor of the soul.

Lee Atwater died, yes. There was no cure for his body, but there was healing for his spirit. His conversion to peace from power, to love from greed, to hope from cynicism, was a greater miracle than a thousand cures. The miracle is always in the healing. If the healing also brings about cure, let us rejoice and be glad. The miracle, however, is in the love.

That's a good definition of miracle, I think: It is the appearance of love where unlove ruled before. Miracle is marked not so much by some otherwise inexplicable phenomenon but by the presence of God. Love, which is the presence of God, is what makes a miracle.

Miracle occurs wherever the *attitude* of triumph, the attitude of love, appears, not any actual event of victory.

Miracle is not about living or dying but about getting whole. Lee Atwater is a miracle.

Sometimes the wholeness of miracle, of love, occurs in the body, sometimes in the spirit, sometimes in both. It is not the cure, however, but the wholeness that writes *miracle* across our lives.

A Roman Catholic priest, Marv Mottet, tells this story of his cancer. I first heard it twenty years ago. I understand it now in a way I couldn't then.

He began to feel weak and went into the hospital for tests. There he first heard that word. The tests showed he had cancer, the incurable kind.

He said, "I walked out with no anger, no discontent. It seemed that a great calmness came over me."

The hospital said there was nothing that could be done for him, no treatment, but that when he got bad enough, they could send him to Houston, where he could be put into an experimental program. He accepted the diagnosis and waited to get worse.

His weakness continued. He could no longer do his regular work. However, he was able to say mass occasionally for a group of cloistered nuns, those who never leave the convent at all but spend all their time in prayer. One of the nuns there, Sister Catherine, told him that she would spend all her time praying for him until he was well. He just smiled; it was a nice gesture.

Finally the cancer had advanced to the point where he could go to the experimental program in Houston. He looked forward to it. By being a guinea pig, he might at least help the researchers learn something that would help other patients. They ran him through all their tests. Then the head researcher called him in.

"Father, why are you here?" he asked.

"Why, because I've got cancer, and they told me when I got bad enough. . . ."

The researcher cut him off with a wave of his test papers. "You don't have cancer, Father, anywhere. We've run every test in the world on you, and you have no cancer at all."

The priest walked out of another hospital, on another street, with the same feeling of calmness that he had felt before, the same calmness both upon hearing he had cancer and upon hearing it had left as mysteriously as it had arrived.

"It was then," he said, "that I realized that in the calendar of saints, it was Saint Catherine's day."

That is a miracle story in several ways, but I am impressed more by the miracle of healing than by the miracle of cure. Please don't misunderstand me. I love cures. I want to be cured. I want you to be cured. The final cure, though, is death. Each of us will die someday, of something. The miracle I see in this story is that calmness of spirit—in diagnosis and weakness, in cure and strength—that same awareness of the presence of God, of the presence of love.

Now that I have cancer, I believe in miracles.

. . . *I steal donkeys.*

"IT'S PALM SUNDAY, SO I want you to go into town and steal me a donkey," Jesus told his disciples. "If anybody catches you, tell them I need it."

Reminds me of the time "Gunner Bob" Rinehart, one of my classmates, happened to notice the keys dangling from the ignition in Mr. Bothwell's new Olds Rocket 88. It was Sunday afternoon, and Gunner decided to take the car for a spin. Mr. Bothwell saw his own car taking off from in front of his house and ran down his driveway after it, house slippers on feet and Sunday funnies in hand.

"Why are you taking my car?" he cried.

Gunner yelled back, "I need it."

You can imagine how much ice that cut with Mr. Bothwell.

One of Jesus' disciples nudged the other as they walked into town and said, "If they go for that, I've got some nice recreational lots along the Dead Sea I can sell them."

All sorts of economists claim Jesus, but he didn't belong to any of them. His approach wasn't economic at all. He just borrowed everything. He borrowed the water he turned into wine and the stone jars from which that wine was poured. He borrowed a boat from which to teach or by which to cross the lake. He borrowed houses in which to eat, teach, and heal. (Some of them did not fare very well, either; one lost its roof so a paralytic could be lowered in to be healed.) He borrowed sons and daughters, brothers and sisters, husbands and wives, to be his disciples. He borrowed the upper room in which he ate his last supper with his borrowed friends. Borrowed was the manger in which he was born, borrowed his cross, and borrowed his tomb.

Jesus is extolled as a giver, not a taker. He was the giver of health, love, truth, and even the ultimate, his own life. Yet Jesus throughout his entire career borrowed things.

This was not just his lifestyle as an itinerant rabbi and philosopher. He was teaching us that all we have is borrowed. He ignored all strictures against lending and borrowing, be it a cloak or a second mile or even one's other cheek, because none of us really has any possessions. Bigger barns, Swiss bank accounts, even gaining the whole world—none of that is enough for us to establish a claim upon ourselves. You yourself, your very life, is borrowed from God, so how can you claim anything you have as your own?

That's why Christians call Jesus "the Word of God." We say he's God's message, God's way of teaching us, God's mouthpiece, if you will. Not just by his words but by his life, he taught us that we do not belong to ourselves but to God.

Gunner and I learned in Sunday School the accounting theory of faith. You get what you have coming to you. Indeed, Gunner got it when he returned Mr. Bothwell's car. One doesn't steal donkeys— or Oldsmobiles—and get away with it in my hometown.

Jesus taught the grace theory, that we are borrowers, that we have no claim on life or God except the one that is given freely, without strings, in love. Grace has no contract requirements, nor can it be attained through manipulation. Grace is what we borrow, knowing we can never repay and knowing that Love the Lender understands that we can never repay.

We cancer patients work at getting well, and so we should. We take chemo and radiation. We visualize and meditate and laugh. That work isn't very useful or effective, however, unless we understand that even it is a gift. The only reason we try to get well is because life is worth living, and the only thing that makes life worth living is love. Why should we get rid of cancer in order to live a life of unlove? But love is always a gift, always borrowed, always grace. By my work I might be able to get you to respect me or fear me or appreciate me or honor me, but there's nothing I can do to get you to love me. Love comes wrapped up, as a present, as something we borrow for a while from the great storehouse of love.

The God of Love comes to us and says, "Borrow from me. Borrow the things that make for life. Let others borrow as well, and do not hinder them. Hell is a life that is earned. Heaven is a life that is borrowed. Borrowed is best. Go steal me a donkey."

Now that I have cancer, I steal donkeys.

. . . *I am broken.*

NOT JUST BROKEN INTO pieces, although that is true in part. Nor am I only broken in spirit, although there's truth there, too. My confidence in my own invincibility is certainly broken. I just never got sick before. Cancer struck other people, not me. There's hardly ever been any cancer in my whole large extended family. Now that confidence, that pride, that arrogance in my own healthiness is broken.

That's not all bad. The Psalmist says, "A broken and a contrite heart, O Lord, you will not despise" (Psalm 51:17). For you see, God uses broken things. That's not all God uses, but God does use broken things.

God uses broken things to create learning. Tommy Lasorda's son died at the age of thirty-three. The longtime Dodger manager said, "If the good Lord had come to me and said, 'I'll give you a son, but you can only have him for thirty-three years, and then your heart will be broken because you'll have to give him back,' I would still have held out my arms and said, 'Hand him over.'"

God uses broken things to create sharing. Jesus broke the bread in order to share it at his last supper, and it could not be shared until it was broken. Reuel Howe tells about a dancing teacher who was paralyzed and in a wheelchair. "I could not teach," she said, "until I was paralyzed. Always before, I was so involved in my own dancing I was unable to share it with anyone else. Now that my body is broken, I can share my dancing."

God uses broken things to create power. Think of the atom. It is simply a tiny particle until it is split. Then, what power! That is in the very nature of things, the way God made the world. The power follows the brokenness.

God uses broken things to create healing. That is seen most easily in the work of an orthopedic surgeon, who often has to break

226

a bone so that it can be reset to heal properly. We cancer patients understand this. We often have to be broken quite literally, have a part of us broken off—a breast or colon or kidney—so that we can be healed.

Oscar Thomas Olson once told this story. As a boy he begged and pleaded for an air rifle, until his father finally bought one for him. One day he was up in the barn loft, shooting his new gun, when he heard the breaking of glass. He remembered that the old-fashioned storm windows from their house—the wooden sash type that are removed in the spring and reinstalled in the fall—were stored in the loft. Sure enough, there they were, piled together in a vertical stack against the wall. The pellet from the air rifle had broken the panes in every window except the last one. Quickly young Oscar Thomas moved the unbroken window to the front of the stack to hide the evidence.

His summer was ruined. He got no joy from his new air rifle. Every day brought him closer to autumn and the day the windows would be brought out to be installed on the house. To make matters worse, his father seemed to go out of his way to brag on him, to tell all their friends and neighbors and relatives what a good boy his son was and how proud he was of him.

Finally the boy could stand it no longer. He went to his father and told him how he had broken all the windows.

"Oh, I knew that," said his father. "I was just waiting for you to tell me."

"I never felt so close to my father in my whole life as I did right then," said Olson.

God uses broken things to bring us back and to bring us close: broken bread, broken relationships, broken bodies.

Now that I have cancer, I am broken, and that's okay.

15. WHEN YOU'RE LOOKING BACK AND FORWARD (EXAMS)

Now that I have cancer . . .

. . . I want to fail my tests.

FOR A CANCER PATIENT, negative is positive. The best news we can get is that there's nothing there. Our top grade is zero.

I suppose cancer patients are the only people in the world who always want to fail their tests. It's the one time *negative* is a good word for us.

"What did the tests show, doc?"

"Nothing."

Now that's a good conversation!

It reminds me of the time Yogi Berra was hit on the head by a fly ball. They took him to the hospital for X-rays. This was the report: "They X-rayed Yogi's head and found nothing." That's funny, of course, especially because it was the strangely philosophical Yogi, but it's also good news. There is often a significant something in the reality of nothingness.

I worry about that nothingness now, because I'm no longer on chemo. The things I'm doing to try to stay well are not medical. There is a comfort in chemotherapy or radiation. Even the side effects we so dread are signs that we are doing something to chase down those speedy little devils. As long as we're doing something, we have some control.

One of my friends lost her beautiful, long red hair during chemo. With treatment over, her hair began to grow back. She said, "It's almost frightening. My baldness was a sign I was actively fighting the cancer. Now I can't help but wonder if anything else is growing back along with my hair."

So we go to our tests with a little bit of fear. What if I don't fail this time? What if there is something instead of nothing?

I don't think there's any way to overcome that fear. We meditate and pray and love and stay busy, but there will always be a little bit of brain that is wondering about those tests.

Perhaps healing is always in absence, in nothingness. Peace of mind, wholeness, happiness—all these depend on being free, of getting to zero. As long as we're lugging a lot of baggage around we're not free. If we depend on the "things" of our lives to give us meaning, we're not yet whole.

That's the exact opposite of how we usually define success, isn't it? Success is getting more, not getting rid of what we've already got. "The one with the most stuff wins." Whether it's money or cars or promotions or victories or sexual partners, the one with the most is the successful one.

Cancer teaches a different lesson about success. The one with the least is the victor.

What did Jesus say? "Go, sell all that you have, and give it to the poor. Then come follow me." It's like the potlatches of some early Native Americans. Instead of having battles where they hit one another with tomahawks and took the spoils of war, they had battles of giving. The tribe that was able to give more was the victor. What a highly civilized way of waging war, and we call them "savage" and "primitive."

It's not just because we've been able to get rid of all our cancer cells that we're victorious. The successful one is the one who fails the hostility test, too, and the nastiness test and the prejudice test and the unkindness test.

I think about Jesus, on his way to Jerusalem, knowing what faced him there. He had to fail his test, too, you know. Think of all the power he had, enough just in the fringe of his robe that it could heal, enough in his vocal cords that he could call Lazarus out of the grave, enough in the soles of his feet that he could walk on water. His test was to *not* use that power, to become a nothing, to stand silent before his accusers, to say, "*Not* my will."

He failed the test. Such a failure is called salvation.

We cancer patients understand that. If we fail our tests, that's good. We know, though, there will come a time when we must fail like Jesus, when we must give up the control, give up the power of chemotherapy and radiation, when the body will give up its existence. That's good, too, because it is part of God's plan to lead us on, to places where these bodies cannot go.

Now that I have cancer, I want to fail my tests.

PART II

WHEN YOU'RE "THOSE WHO LOVE THEM"

16. WHEN HOPE BECOMES ROUTINE

(LONG-TERM SURVIVING)

Now that I'm a long-term survivor . . .

. . . I face the dailyness of it.

WINSTON CHURCHILL SAID THERE is no feeling more exhilarating than being shot at without results. I know that feeling. I dodged the cancer bullet. It exhilarated me. I never felt more alive, even in the midst of fear and misery, than when I was fighting cancer.

But you can't live on the edge all the time. There's a time to go sky-diving and a time to get back to earth and go to work.

There's an interesting story about Jesus called "The Transfiguration." He takes his closest friends, they go up on the mountain, and they have an experience of God. Jesus is transfigured right before the eyes of his friends, and they see Moses and Elijah, too. They say, "This is great. Let's stay up here on the mountain." But Jesus says, "No. Back down in the plain space is where the action is." He leads them down, and sure enough, people are waiting for them with the nitty-gritty problem of a sick child, the dailyness of Jesus' life. (You can read about it in Matthew 17:1–8, Mark 9:2–8, or Luke 9:28–36.)

My favorite author is Elaine Fowler Palencia, and one of her books of poetry is *The Dailyness of It.* It's her attempt to communicate with her son, Andrew, even though he can never read it. He is in his thirties now. He has multiple problems with his body and brain. He needs constant care. He has never spoken.

Reading Elaine about the dailyness of dealing with Andrew reminds me that most of life is lived in the routine of dailyness. If we find joy and meaning only in the occasional periods of intensity and excitement, most of life will be wasted.

Many years ago I read a novel that featured an inventor who had created a "happiness machine." You sat in it and all your cares melted away. At first, everyone in his family and in the neighborhood came to sit in the happiness machine. Then they stopped coming. He couldn't understand why. He complained to his wife about it.

"What you don't understand," she said, "is that a person can't be happy all the time. You go inside that machine and sure, the air smells good all the time and nobody bothers you and everything is fine. But you come back out, and there are dirty dishes waiting."

Later that night he came up the front walk of his house. It was dark outside and the lights were on. He saw his wife fixing supper in the kitchen, his daughter doing her homework, his sons playing a board game. He looked into his own home and thought, "Ah, there it is, the happiness machine."

Now that I have survived, I am whole in the dailyness of it.

. . . *I still need good examples.*

AS I MENTIONED IN the *Introduction,* a woman called our house a few years ago looking for a copy of the first edition of this book. My wife answered the phone and assured the woman that the book was available, but she seemed reluctant to commit to buying it. She asked a number of questions about me. Finally she said, "I just wanted to be sure he was still alive before I bought the book."

It's a bit strange, in a way. After all, people still get a lot out of *The Letter to the Romans,* and *Ethics,* and *Hamlet,* even though Paul of Tarsus and Aristotle and Shakespeare are no longer alive. On the other hand, I don't blame her. If you are dealing with cancer, you want all the good examples you can find, and long-term survivors are good examples.

As I write this, my younger sister is taking the second round of chemotherapy for ovarian cancer. She was not given a good prognosis at diagnosis, but she is beginning to meet survivors who were given similar prognoses and are going strong ten years later. She says, "I figure, why not me? I might as well be in that group."

I remember that feeling well. Careless words by my first oncologist made me think I would be dead within two years. Then I began to meet long-term survivors. "Oh, yes. I had colon cancer twenty years ago." Twenty years? Wow! That's a whole lot more than two.

It has been thirty-five years since Lynn Ringer, the co-founder of CanSurmount, survived ovarian cancer when the survival rate was only 1 percent. In the summer of my year of chemotherapy, Helen and I took a course at Iliff Theological Seminary on "Empowering the Cancer Patient," Lynn was one of the teachers.

At that time, she was a twenty-year survivor. Most of us were pastors in training, but also there was one patient and a couple of spouses of patients. One day as we sat around our circle, John Anduri asked each of us, "Where do you want to be in twenty years?" My response was, "I want to be sitting in Lynn's chair, telling the same story she tells." I'm almost there. I like being a good example.

On the other hand, Dana Reeve is an awfully good example of how to deal with cancer, not because she was a long survivor, not because she was cured, but because she was whole. She spent almost her whole adult life caring for her quadriplegic husband, Christopher Reeve. After his death, she had hardly any time at all to catch her breath and do something for herself before her own cancer diagnosis, treatment, and death. She lived her life, with or without cancer, in wholeness. Life is not measured by years on the calendar nearly so much as by years in the heart. By that measure, she lived a full life.

I really thought that if I got more years after cancer, I would never waste a moment of them. I would appreciate every pain-free minute, live in each moment, embrace every opportunity, live only in love. But you know what? I accept pain-free minutes as my right. I waste all kinds of time that I could be using for good deeds. I make silly mistakes.

I still need good examples. They don't have to be long-term survivors. They just need to be folks who know how to appreciate each moment, who know the way to wholeness.

Now that I'm a survivor, I still need good examples.

. . . *You owe me.*

IF YOU ARE GETTING chemo for colon cancer, you owe me. I'm the guy who did twelve months on the clinical trial to prove you need only six months. A whole lot of bad things happened to me in those last six months. They won't happen to you because you don't have to do those extra six months. You owe me!

When Dr. Hatfield told me there really was something I could do after surgery besides look over my shoulder to see whether those little cockeyed, bowlegged, mouth-breathing cancer characters were gaining on me, I was relieved. For fifteen minutes. Then I found out it was a clinical trial. The computer would randomly select some patients for six months of hell and some for twelve. I knew the minute he said it that the computer would sentence me to twelve months. Computers feel that way about me.

When I got to three months, I didn't think I would make it even to six. I had every side effect that chemo ever caused. I was miserable. One morning about 2 A.M., I promised myself that if I got to six months, I could quit. Then I made the mistake of telling Alan Hatfield I was switching to the six-month group.

My doctor was not very sympathetic. "You'll mess up the results of the clinical trial," he screamed. "How will we know whether to give future patients six months or twelve?"

"I don't care about future patients," I yelled. "I care about one current patient, and he's miserable!"

Actually, I didn't yell that. It was what I thought, but it sounded really selfish, so I didn't say it out loud. Instead, I gritted my teeth and anything else I could grit, and I gritted it out.

Because I knew I owed every one who had taken the journey before me, every patient and doctor and nurse and pharmacist and researcher who had contributed to the pool of knowledge and compassion into which each patient dips the bucket of hope and healing.

There are people who spend long years earning degrees in chemistry or biology and then don long white coats and disappear for years behind rows of test tubes in windowless laboratories until they emerge with thinning hair and blurry eyes and a new drug that just might smite a blastoma or a melanoma or some other oma.

Other people spend years in medical or nursing or pharmacy schools to learn how to apply what the researchers find.

And you and me, sister, you and me, brother—we're the human guinea pigs, the ones who do the six months or twelve on a clinical trial to make the way a little easier for those who come after us.

All who come after us owe us, but we owe the ones who went before. The cancer family is a big bunch of debtors. Each of us owes, and each of us is owed.

If you've done only six months of chemo, remember just *who* it is to whom you owe the most.

Now that I'm a long-term survivor, you owe me.

. . . *I'm in the big story.*

WHEN I WAS A kid, I wanted to be a newspaper reporter. Not the kind who wrote about what happened at the city council meeting but the kind who got "the big story." That was the name of a radio show I listened to each week. It dramatized how different reporters got their big story. A big story was always one that dealt with people, with life and death, usually with pulling life out of death. But I was derailed from the newspaper track by a "strange calling" to be a pastor. (You can read about that in *The Strange Calling: Stories of Ministry,* published by Smyth & Helwys.)

I did not give up writing, though. I wrote a lot of published pieces on that big story subject of life and death—short stories, articles, sermons. *Now That I Have Cancer, I Am Whole* was my first book, however.

I think my family, including aunts and uncles and cousins but especially my wife and children and sons-in-law, got even more enjoyment out of telling people about the first edition of this book than I did. Some of them even went into bookstores to be sure that the cover was turned face out, and if it was not, they assisted the bookstore with subtle rearrangements to make the book more noticeable.

My daughters told a young woman friend about my book, and one day she related this story: "Six months ago, I had a test for AIDS. It came back positive. They told me sometimes they got false positives, but they had to wait six months before they could test again to be sure. I knew I had done things that made it possible for me to get AIDS. I knew if I had it I was under a death sentence. I felt so scared and alone. I was so ashamed I couldn't tell my friends. I certainly couldn't tell my parents. I couldn't tell anybody. But you had talked so much about your father's book, about how good it was, about how proud you were. I figured if it was good for cancer patients, maybe it would be good for an AIDS patient, too. For six months, it was my only companion in my loneliness. I just had the test again. The first one was a false positive. I'm okay. But I'm so thankful you bragged so much about your dad's book. It was my support group of one."

I understood what she meant. When I was too sick or tired to go to support group, I read or listened to tapes. The authors of those books were my support group. I have a friend who hands copies of this book to patients and says, "Here's your support group." I'll always be grateful that my own big story became a support group for that young woman who thought she might have AIDS. I hope it's part of your support group, too.

Now that I'm a long-term survivor, I'm in the big story, a support group of one, one with everyone else who's in the story.

. . . I live in Philadelphia.

HAVE YOU SEEN THE movie *Philadelphia*? In it Tom Hanks plays young lawyer Andrew Beckett, who is homosexual, gets AIDS, and is fired from his firm. The partners claim they fired him for poor performance, but until they knew of his AIDS and homosexuality, he was the golden boy, consistently rated as the best. He sued the firm and won. Along the way we saw him in relationships with his lover, his mother, his friends, his colleagues.

The film was a must-see and won many awards, including an Oscar for "Best Actor" for Hanks and a nomination for screenwriter Ron Nyswaner.

The movie was released shortly after the publication of the first edition of this book. Someone sent me a copy of a review of the movie when it came out. In a Philadelphia newspaper, the reviewer said, "When I came out of the theater, someone asked me what I thought about it, and I said the first thing that came to my mind: 'It's a commercial for AIDS.' We've gotten to where we are identified by our diseases. I mean, look at this new book, *Now That I Have Cancer, I Am Whole.*"

I was stunned. I thought, "Oh, good grief! Did I miss something? Is my book a commercial for cancer? Am I saying that we are identified by this disease, cancer? Did I do the exact opposite of what I intended to?"

I have heard two criticisms of the first edition of *Now That I Have Cancer, I Am Whole.* A friend gave it to a cancer patient who read it and said dryly, "He's a good deal too optimistic for me." I regret that she could not be more optimistic, but there is little I can do about that.

I have heard the second criticism several times: "You don't have to have cancer to be whole."

I happily agree. I do not mean to speak for anyone but myself when I say, "Now that I have cancer, I am whole." The joyful and difficult struggle toward wholeness is what life is all about for anyone, regardless of cancer. But for those of us who *are* cancer survivors, there is no way to get whole outside of cancer. It is our particular doorway to wholeness, our chance to be healed regardless of whether we are cured.

I think the movie reviewer got it wrong. *Philadelphia* is not a commercial for AIDS; it is a commercial for love. It tries to say that love is the point of life, and love can triumph even in the face of death. Likewise, this book is not a commercial for cancer. It is a commercial for healing. It tries to say that we can be whole, even in the face of brokenness.

Philadelphia means "city of brotherly love." Brotherly or any other kind, cancer gives us the chance not to concentrate on a disease but on love.

Now that I have cancer, I live in the city of love.

. . . I get reminders that I might get it again.

A SMALL, HARD PYRAMID of flesh appeared on my left temple. I'm a little old for pimples, and it was too hard for a pimple anyway. I took it, along with the rest of me, to my family physician. "It's probably nothing," he said, "but I'll remove it and send it to the lab." A few days later he called. "It's a squamous cell skin cancer," he said. "Let's send you to the dermatologist."

The dermatologist looked me over, said he couldn't find anything else that looked suspicious, gave me a lecture about staying out of the sun, and told me to keep coming back for regular appointments.

My chemo for the colon cancer made me sun-sensitive, so I've been wearing long sleeves and big brims for fifteen years anyway. The problem is that I started too late. I'm a blond. (Well, I *was* a blond.) I grew up on a farm. Every summer I worked with my shirt off. Every summer I got a deep tan, starting with a bad burn. Couple that background with the eroding ozone layer, and I know that I have a good shot at more skin cancers.

Of course, there are the regular colonoscopies of what my proctologist calls my "tortuous" semicolon. (I think that means it twists and turns a lot.)

And every week some friend calls and announces she or he has cancer of one sort or another.

There are reminders every day that I'm not free of the threat of cancer, ever. Your reminders may be different from mine, but that is true for you, too. The threat is always there, and the trigger that makes the cancer possible may be something long in the past, like my farmer's sunburns.

I can't do anything about those sunburns now, though. I can't do anything about whatever it was that caused my colon cancer, either. But I don't think that means it's okay to sit out in the sun and eat barbecued ribs on the theory that the damage has already been done.

The life I have to live, to enjoy, and to protect, is the one I have starting right now. I'm not going to waste any of it on worry every time a reminder comes along that I might get cancer again. But neither am I going to ignore the things I can do now to protect myself from a recurrence of cancer.

Taking cancer precautions is just a fact of life these days. So I accept the reminders that I need to be careful. I accept them as reminders that right now is the time to live in joy.

Now that I'm a survivor, I get reminders that I might get cancer again, reminders to live in joy.

. . . *I know the purpose of life is to have a good time.*

I THINK THAT'S WHAT Jesus of Nazareth meant when he said, "I'm here; let's party." John 10:10 usually is translated, "I have come that they may have life and have it abundantly," but I think "I'm here; let's party" is even better.

The opposite of a good time is not a bad time. Cancer is a bad time, but that does not mean it can't be a good time, too. Any time that helps us to become whole, that gives us joy, is a good time.

Many people recoil at the idea of life's purpose being "merely" a good time. But there is nothing "mere" about a good time.

I'm not talking about the stupid things we do and then say, "But I had a good time." Those are false good times. That's the opposite of a good time. It's partial instead of whole, fool's gold instead of real gold, pleasure instead of joy.

The shorthand way to tell a true good time from a false good time is this: A true good time feels bad in the short run but is good for you in the long run. A false good time feels good now but produces problems later. Chemotherapy feels bad now. So does exercise. So does going without an extra helping. But they give us the promise of health. Smoking and drinking and drugs and sugar and recreational sex feel good at the moment but produce illness and dis-ease later.

There is *pleasure* in false good times. We wouldn't pursue false good times if we did not get pleasure. Jesus of Nazareth understood that. He said of those willing to settle for pleasure in place of joy, "They have their reward." Sure they do. We wouldn't get drunk or high or take a chance on AIDS or gambling the mortgage away if we didn't get some pleasure from it.

One of the worst things about pleasure is that it makes us think it is better than joy, or at least an adequate substitute. Some wag said, "Money can't buy love, but it can buy sex, and that's just as good." No, it's not, but love is hard and takes work. All sex takes is a fistful of dollars or someone else who is just as desperate for love but willing to settle for sex, hoping for joy but willing to settle for pleasure.

There are many forces around us that try to make us think pleasure is an adequate substitute for joy: advertisers who want us to buy their products, people who want us to satisfy their sexual desires, people who want us to do stupid things so they won't feel alone in their stupidity or so they can feel superior, people who appeal to our fear and hate so that we'll vote for them.

Pleasure is not necessarily bad. I get pleasure from sipping iced tea on the patio on a hot summer evening. There's nothing wrong with that, but when the woman who has always loved me and always will comes out and sits down with me and holds my hand, then I am my true self. I am whole; I receive joy.

Joy does not necessarily depend on the presence of other people. It often comes in relationships, because joy is in wholeness, in connections. Sometimes, though, none of the relationships that might be carriers of joy are available to us. People we love may be dead or gone, but that does not mean we cannot be our true selves.

I think of someone like John McCain in a prison cell in Vietnam. Politically, I have a number of disagreements with Senator McCain, but I admire him because, even in his worst moments in that cell, he had a good time. Pleasure was totally absent, but he had joy because he was true to what he knew was right. He was his own true self.

Sometimes when we have cancer, we are in an isolated cell of pain. It's a bad time, but we can still have a good time.

Pleasure is just that: pleasure. Joy is much more than pleasure. Joy is fulfillment, being who we are really meant to be, wholeness, love.

> *Now that I'm a long-term survivor, I know that the purpose of life is to have a good time.*

. . . *I am brave.*

IN A MEDICAL SETTING, a patient's primary concern is "Am I safe here? Do I have anything to fear?" Our fears arise either because we do not know the answer or because we do. If we have any fears at all, facing a doctor or disease or diagnosis will call them out into the light.

Fear has been the dominant emotion, perhaps the dominant reality, of my life. I grew up in a chaotic home. I'm sure our parents loved my siblings and me as best they could, but they were consistently inconsistent, often abusive, sometimes violent, always frightening.

"Where courage is absent, no other virtue is possible, except by accident." Samuel Johnson said that. I read it as a teenager. It caused me a great deal of grief because I knew I was not a person of courage. I was a person of fear, and so I was doomed to a life without virtue.

Many of my friends and acquaintances will be surprised to learn of my fears, for they have usually seen me as a brave person. That is because, in my desperate attempt to be a real person, I became the opposite of real. I became a fake.

I began to fake courage. I pretended. I acted brave when I was really scared to the ends of my fingernails.

I don't mean the silly kind of fake courage—jumping into shallow water from a high cliff, or challenging the meanest guy in the bar to a fight. Not even refusing to buckle my seat belt or riding a bicycle without a helmet. It's not surprising that since I was so afraid of the power figures in my family, my parents, I tried to fake courage by standing up to power figures in other places.

As a high school student I challenged the principal and teachers on actions or rules I thought were unfair. Later I marched in civil rights demonstrations. I have called liars liars, even if they were mayors or congressmen or board chairs or deans or bishops. I ignored what would be best for my career in favor of speaking the truth. That was not because I was brave; it was because I *wanted* to be brave.

Then I got cancer. I was face to face with surgery, recovery, and twelve months of chemo, and, most importantly, the ultimate and most fearsome authority figure: death. To my surprise and amazement, I did not have to fake the courage this time. It was there. I really believed what I had been faking—that truth makes us free, that love conquers death. I was, in C. S. Lewis's felicitous phrase, "surprised by joy." I could honestly say, "*Now that I have cancer, I am whole.*" I was finally real.

Or maybe not. I know it sounds incredibly naïve, but I really thought the battle was over. No more fear. I had faced the worst that fear could serve up and knocked it out of the ring with the sword of wholeness. Obviously, overcoming fear did not overcome the desire to use terrible mixed metaphors.

Survival was going to be a breeze. I was finally whole, and now I would have no more fears, only joys. Problems, sure. They come with life. But I would no longer cringe in front of them. I would just grab them by the hair and pummel them into submission. Problems would not be fears.

You know, it didn't work out that way. I survived, yes, and so did the fears. They were still out there, lying in wait, their beady little eyes peeking up out of the ditch, just waiting for my unsuspecting ankles to come skipping along, and they have grabbed me and tripped me more than once.

Now that I had cancer, I was whole, I was real, but I was still the same fearful little boy I had always been and apparently always will be.

"Where courage is absent, no other virtue is possible." That does not mean that fear and courage cannot exist together. That was the mistake I made. I assumed being a person of courage meant I would have *no* fear, but fear and courage walk hand in hand through this life. In fact, they depend on each other. We don't recognize one without the other.

> *Now that I have survived, I am whole, and I'm afraid, and I am brave.*

17. WHEN THE GENERATIONS ARE UPSIDE DOWN

(A PARENT OR SIBLING IS THE PATIENT)

Now that I'm the child
and brother of cancer patients . . .

. . . I'm a cancer fashion leader.

AT A TIME WHEN 56 percent of men and 42 percent of women get cancer (NCI), my extended family of McFarlands and Ponds has a remarkable health record. Only one of my thirteen aunts and uncles has had cancer, and Aunt Ginny was ninety when diagnosed. None of my twenty-eight cousins has had cancer, nor have any of their children.

My immediate family spoils the record, and it's all my fault. I made it possible; I was the first. Since I broke the dam, my brother, father, mother, grandson, wife, younger sister, and older daughter have been swept into the cancer river.

There is interesting speculation and some research about the relationship between a person's position in the family and the onset of cancer. It's possible that who gets it first makes a difference. There may be opinion leaders in health as well as in fashion. Birth order is part of it, but so is your role, whether you're the "good" child, the black sheep, or the overachiever, and so on.

So when I say that the almost total incidence of cancer in my immediate family is all my fault, I have to wonder whether there's some truth in that beyond the simple fact that I was first. Why have so many in my nuclear family gotten cancer when almost no one in our extended family has? Why did no one else get it, even my parents, until I did? I know I'm a fashion leader, but is there such a thing as a cancer leader?

I've known Paul Unger since he was twenty. As we age, he blames me for all his ills. "You started it," he says. "You opened the gates by getting cancer. Now all of your friends are getting sick, too." Paul is serious only about half the time, and his wife, Judith, says it's a lot less than that, but there is always a kernel of wisdom even in his jolly jests. We are individuals, but we affect one another in surprising ways. Illness can be catching for more reasons than passing germs along.

My friend and once next-door neighbor Bob Teague thought so. I still remember that telephone call. "I've always admired you," he said, "and I wanted to be like you, but I've taken it too far. Now I've got cancer, just like you."

Did Bob really get cancer because of my example? Probably not, not exactly, but he knew we had a connection and that it was important.

So what does this mean? I'm not sure. I do know that I'm glad I was the first in my family, and among my friends, to step into the cancer waters, because it gives me a chance to be the first to use cancer as a safety vest, as a way to swim to shore, as a way to get whole. I can model not only how to wear many plaids at the same time but how to get well, with or without a cure. Being first may have been a curse I put on my family, but it was also a gift I was able to give, even to my parents. I may have opened the floodgates to cancer, but I had the chance to open the doors to hope, too.

Now that I am the child of cancer people, I have a special gift to give.

. . . I see backward.

MY MOTHER WAS A contrarian. Some folks are just that way.

I recall a couple in a church I pastored. I'll call them Bob and Connie. For some reason they got the idea that people were trying to drive them out of the church. They made an appointment to call me on the phone. I made sure that my secretary, Mary Putney, listened on the extension. Bob had Connie on the extension at their house.

"Is it true that you don't want Connie to be president of the women's group at church?" he asked.

"No, not at all," I said. "We value the presence of both of you. We definitely want Connie to be president of the women's group."

"Well, it's clear they don't want us, Connie," Bob snorted.

"Yes, isn't it," Connie sniffed.

They hung up and never returned to church.

I wandered into Mary's office. She shrugged her shoulders, which was the only appropriate response.

Now, I suppose Bob and Connie might have thought being president of the women's group was cruel and unusual punishment, and you would do that only to someone you wanted to drive out. But I don't think so. I think they were just contrarians. They wanted so much to be victims that they heard whatever they needed to in order to play that role.

That brings us back to Mother. The cancer of a parent brings to the surface all sorts of feelings and fears. It's not just the advance of the generations, the awareness that when our parents are gone, we no longer have a buffer against our own mortality. It's the unfinished business that we were able to ignore as long as we thought our parents would live forever. Most parent–child relationships have unresolved feelings. A parent's cancer reminds us that our time for dealing with those is limited.

When my mother went to the hospital for the last time, it was clearly time for her to get out of a body that was no longer an adequate place to live. The doctor knew that. My wife knew it. I did not. I lost my head. I insisted the doctor try a blood transfusion that everyone else knew was useless.

I spent my life trying to make my mother happy and received nothing but frustration in return. Most of my life I longed to be free of the burdens she heaped upon me, but when the time for freedom came, I could not let go. As long as she was alive, there was a chance I might finally understand her and find a way to make her happy.

Mother's grave did not have a stone for seven years. The plan was to wait until Dad died and then erect a common stone over their graves. After Dad's funeral, the stone was put in place, but it was several months before Helen and I were at the cemetery at Forsythe Church to see it.

It was backward! Every other stone in the whole line faced one way, and my parents' stone faced the other.

It's tempting to think the stone setters knew my mother and were just doing the logical thing. I suspect it was more incompetence than intention, though. Still, somebody finally got something right for mother, something that would make her happy. She could face the opposite way forever!

That backward gravestone is a touchstone for me. I finally understand my mother. She did the best she could. It was just that she could not see the needs of anyone else because she was always looking in the other direction.

Now that I'm the child of cancer people, I can accept them for who they are.

. . . *I still don't prepare.*

WHEN CHRIS SCHILLIG, THE editorial director of Andrews McMeel, e-mailed me to say they wanted to publish a new edition of this book, I was not prepared, even though I was the one who had suggested it in the first place. The reason is simple: I *still* don't prepare. (There is a different meditation titled "I don't prepare" in Part I of this book.)

The reason I don't prepare anymore is simple, too. It's my father's fault.

When Mother died, Dad moved to a senior citizen apartment building and quickly became very popular with the ladies. The reasons for that were simple, too. First, there are not many men in those places. Second, my father was a very handsome man, as you might guess from my picture on the back cover.

Dad was ninety, and when I discussed his popularity with the ladies with him, he just dismissed it with "I don't know what it is, but I guess I've got it."

Whatever it was, he was soon "keeping company," quite literally, with Betty, from next door. At seventy-two, she was the proverbial younger woman. After breakfast, she came to his apartment to listen to music. (Dad was blind, so they did not watch TV.) Then they went to her apartment for lunch. After lunch, back to his apartment for more music and supper, then to hers for dessert, and back to his for more music.

Once, when my wife and I went to visit him, he called us at the inn where we were staying and said, "I want you to come in early today, before Betty gets here. There's something I want to discuss with you."

Well, we knew what *that* was. He was going to tell us he wanted to marry Betty, and that would create all sorts of problems, particularly with my sisters. So Helen got on the phone and called all the necessary offices to find out what happens to finances and such when old people get married. I called Len Kirkpatrick, our state police trooper "son," to find out how to find a private detective to check Betty out. He's not really our son, but he thinks he is, and sometimes it's good to have a cop in the family, so we let him keep thinking it.

When we got there, Dad said, "Well, I suppose you know what I want to talk with you about."

"Yes," we said, "we know."

"That's right. When your brother and I sell that house we own, I want to pay you that six thousand dollars your little sister owes you."

There was a very long silence while Helen and I gulped a lot. Finally I said, "You want to pay what Margey owes?"

"Yes. She wants to, but she's had too many setbacks. She'll never be able to do it."

"You don't want to marry Betty?"

"Marry Betty? Why would I want to marry Betty? What part of *I want to give you money* don't you understand?"

We had spent all morning getting ready for something that didn't happen.

But we were going to get money! Helen started making plans for a screened-in porch. I started looking at red pickup trucks. Then the house deal fell through, and we didn't get the money. We had spent all *that* time getting ready for porches and pickups that weren't going to happen.

The stuff I prepare for never happens. What happens is the stuff I don't expect to happen. So there's no point in preparing for stuff because it takes time away from preparing your self.

I don't prepare for stuff that might happen, but I do prepare myself. I prepare my soul. I prepare my life. I get whole. It's a lifelong process, getting whole, but it's the only preparation that matters.

> *Now that I'm in a cancer family, I don't prepare for what might happen, but I prepare the one to whom it will happen.*

. . . *We are a backward family.*

MY FATHER INHERITED COLON cancer from me. In other words, I got it first, three years before he did.

His tumor was close enough to the rectum that most surgeons we consulted said he would have to have a permanent colostomy. That's a difficult thing for a blind man, especially one who is already the nurse for his wife. We looked around and found a surgeon who said he could do the surgery in such a way that Dad would have a temporary colostomy, but he could reverse it in two months. That sounded better. Better still, that surgeon was at a hospital just twenty miles from where we lived.

Or maybe that was not better, because my parents had to live with us while my father had the surgeries.

We knew it was a mistake, but there was no choice. I think it was "only" three months. It felt like three years, or three decades.

My mother lived in her own world. She did not much care for the one in which everyone else lived, and she never passed up an opportunity to express her discontent with it. She also insisted that everyone else adjust their world to accommodate hers. That is always hard to accomplish, so Mother was hardly ever happy, with anyone or anything.

One day the hospital called and said they were ready to release Dad, but someone in the family had to take colostomy training first.

Helen's brother-in-law John Decker started in the medical department at Inland Steel as an ambulance driver. He worked his way up and is now the administrative head of the department. In his first year, there was a bad accident at the mill. John grabbed the doctor and the ambulance and raced to the building where the accident happened. He jumped out, grabbed all the equipment, and got ready to run to the scene, only to find the doctor standing beside the ambulance, smoking a cigarette.

"Come on, Doc," John said. "We've got to hurry."

"I don't know, John," the doctor replied. "I'm no blood and guts man."

I know just how he felt. I would have made a great doctor, except for the blood and guts and colostomies.

"What do you mean, colostomy training?" I yelled at the voice on the phone. "You said the visiting nurses would take care of that!"

"They will, but we can't release him until someone in the family has colostomy training, and we want to release him *now*, so someone has to come for colostomy training *now*."

Well, that was okay. Helen could do it. It is a truly stupid man who does not marry a woman smarter than he. Then, when there is a hard or difficult job to do, the wife does it because she knows it is the only way it will be done right. That is the way it has always been in our family. I get out of all the bad jobs because Helen is so much better at them. But my smart wife could not do this. She was in her classroom. There was no one to go for colostomy training but me.

I admire men who are able and willing to cry, but that has always been difficult for me. Nonetheless, I was on the edge of tears, the very close and steep edge. It wasn't just the prospect of colostomy training, of course, that put me on the verge of tears. It was the accumulated stress of worrying about Dad and dealing with Mother.

I told Mother that I had to go to the hospital for colostomy training, that I would be bringing Dad home, that I would fix lunch when we returned but that there was stuff in the refrigerator in case she got hungry.

I was drooping out of the house, trying to hold back the tears, when my mother called after me, "Did I ever tell you what an ugly baby you were?"

She wasn't trying to be mean. It was just something she thought of, and so she said it, like everything else she ever thought of. It really was not the thing I needed to hear right then.

In a way, it didn't bother me, because it wasn't true. I have seen pictures of me as a baby; I was quite cute! But it *did* bother me, of course, both for my sake and for hers. Was I such a bad son that she recalled me as an ugly baby when I was not? Had Mother's soul become so warped that she recalled everything as ugly, even the son who spent his life, not just the few months she lived in our house, trying so hard to make her life better?

Helen was always an amazingly gracious daughter-in-law. She and I did the best we could for Mother. We spent time with her. We listened to her. We took her to appointments and shopping and out to eat. We gave her gifts, even though she criticized them and refused to use or wear them.

Mother died of chronic lymphocytic leukemia when she was eighty-seven. I spent my life trying to make her happy. Helen shared in that quest for thirty-seven years. We never succeeded, because that is impossible. None of us can make someone else happy.

That is a major concern for us when a family member has cancer. We want to make life better for them, or at least easier. We want to make them happy. But we cannot give anyone the gift of attitude. That is something each of us chooses by and for ourselves.

We cannot give the gift of attitude, but we can give the gift of ourselves. We can do all we can to be of help. Even if that does not make our parent or spouse or child or friend happy, it is all we can do. It is enough, even if it is not enough, because it is all we have.

I was an ugly baby to my mother, and I was not able
to make her happy, but I was a good son.

18. WHEN YOU ARE IN THE SUICIDE SEAT

(A SPOUSE IS THE PATIENT)

Now that my wife has cancer . . .

. . . I don't trust cameras or hair.

GEORGE FOREMAN IS A good friend of mine. Actually, I met him only once, in the briefest of ways, but George has a way of making you think he's been your friend forever and making you want to buy a grill. But he's an even closer friend to Helen.

We met George in Houston, where I spoke at an M.D. Anderson patient conference. It was a great conference. I had corresponded for years with Cindy Melancon, who started *Conversations,* the newsletter for ovarian cancer patients, and we finally got to meet her in person. Other speakers were Wendy Harpham, M.D., and Steve Allen Jr., also M.D., and Scott Burton, the comedian and juggler. All of them were delightful. George was there too, and he explained that he named all his children, male and female, George Foreman Jr. because, as he put it, "You wouldn't expect me to name them after Muhammad Ali, would you?"

Judy Gerner was the director of the M.D. Anderson Network then. Judy is tall, beautiful, and unflappable. The unflappable part came in handy when she tried to get George from the doors of the hotel ballroom past all the tables and up to the stage.

As soon as they entered the room, people jumped up and ran to George. He smiled and shook hands and slapped backs. All the while, Judy had him by the arm, pulling him steadily toward the dais. The crowd around him swirled like a small dust cloud. Most amazing to me, my wife was in that crowd.

Helen is the world's most intelligent woman but its least knowledgeable sports fan. She thinks the third base coach makes those signs because he is Catholic. She refers to uniforms as costumes. She insists that a football player cannot run around his own end. Our daughters and I once had a dozen of her teacher pencils specially imprinted so that if any of her high school students asked a sports question, she could casually glance at her pencil and say, "The Lakers play basketball."

Was this gentle woman a closet boxing fan? There she was, circling George with the rest of the crowd, her camera in front of her face, snapping pictures from north, south, east, and west.

Judy finally broke George free, and Helen returned to our table. I looked at her in astonishment.

"I didn't know you even knew who George Foreman is, but you must have taken a dozen pictures of him," I said.

"Who? Oh, that nice man with Judy? I wasn't taking pictures of him. When we get home, I want my hairdresser to fix my hair like Judy's, so I thought I'd take advantage of the commotion to get some pictures of Judy's hair."

What you see is not always what you get. Eyewitnesses are not that reliable. There were three hundred people in that room who would tell you to this day that the nice lady with the tall bearded guy was taking pictures of George Foreman. They say the camera doesn't lie, but Helen's camera certainly deceived people.

Wendy Harpham told this story at that conference: Two hunters were shooting at ducks. One shot ten feet in front of the duck. One shot ten feet behind the duck. On average, the duck was dead.

We don't live by averages. We don't live by theories. We don't live by appearances. We live by stories, which are often told in song, because story and song allow us to hear and tell the truth in ways that averages and outward appearances don't.

Don't trust the averages and percentages. Don't trust appearances. Don't trust theories. Trust love, which sees with the eyes of the heart.

I see Helen with heart as well as eyes. She looked great before Judy's hairdo. She looked great with Judy's hairdo. She looked great when she was bald from chemo. She looks great now with the salt-and-pepper hair that never waved before chemo but does so nicely now.

Someday I'll tell you about the time Helen held hands with Walter Payton on a street in Champaign, Illinois. She even knew who he was. Sort of. "I understand why they call him Sweetness, but what does he do?"

Now that I'm in the suicide seat, I don't trust cameras to tell the story, but I do trust love.

. . . *I get morloved.*

I JUST HAD THE greatest idea for a meditation for this book. I mean, it was perfect. And I was just ready to write it down when I forgot it.

Not all by myself. I got porlocked.

Helen walked into the room and said something or asked me something or did something. I'm not sure what it was, but she *porlocked* me. By the time I dealt with the something, that fantastic, world-changing idea for a meditation was as gone as the last three hundred lines of Samuel Taylor Coleridge's poem about Kubla Khan.

Here's Coleridge's story of how he got *porlocked*. He awoke from a dream with the entire poem written, right in front of his eyes, three or four hundred lines. He feverishly started grabbing it out of the air and putting it down on paper. "In Xanadu did Kubla Khan a stately pleasure dome decree. . . . " He had written only a few lines when "a person from Porlock" came and knocked on his door and tried to sell him a horse or something. By the time he got back to his pen and inkpot, the poet could remember only fifty or sixty lines of the original.

I used to be very thankful to the person from Porlock because Mr. Herman Cloin made me memorize "Kubla Khan" in sophomore English, and I was *glad* it did not have four hundred lines. That was before I got porlocked by Helen. Now the world is deprived of the chance to read my riveting prose about whatever it was.

Helen has been porlocking me from the very beginning. I always had this thing for wiry little brunettes, especially in college. I was just about to put the moves on a wiry little brunette one day when this sweet, soft blonde appeared. I forgot all about three hundred or so other girls, just as Coleridge forgot three hundred lines of his poem. I was porlocked forever.

I don't know how many times Helen has porlocked me. I know it happens several times a day, though. I'm thinking some great thought, and she comes into view, and I just can't think about anything but her.

When the doctor said Helen had cancer, that was a porlock moment. There wasn't anything else worth thinking about. You know, it wasn't the cancer, or the possibility of separation by death, that grabbed my consciousness. I considered all the great thoughts she had porlocked and knew that all together they did not add up to a single moment of being with her. She was not the Person from Porlock. She was the Person from Morlove.

The next time someone you love interrupts you in the middle of something you think is important, take a good look at that person. Whatever it was that got interrupted is *not* that important. Thank God you have someone who loves you enough to porlock you. That is the Person from Morlove.

Now that I'm the husband of a survivor, I get morloved.
I'm glad.

. . . I know the rule of friendship.

THERE ARE UNWRITTEN RULES about everything.

There's nothing in the baseball rule book that says if one of your teammates is knocked down by "a high, hard one" from the opposing pitcher, your pitcher has to knock down someone from his team, too. But that's a rule less flexible than "three strikes and you're out," even though it's not in the rule book or "Take Me Out to the Ball Game."

There are unwritten rules about where and when you can talk to strangers. For instance, there's no "stranger talking" if you're standing at a row of urinals. However, it's okay to talk to a stranger at a bookstore if the subject is books, coffee, or music. At my favorite bookstore, Larry Dunphy's Books on First, the rule is expanded to include almost any subject.

One day I was chatting with a woman about T-shirts.

"This kid was wearing a T-shirt that said 'You don't want to know what I'm thinking,'" she told me. "I asked him why I didn't want to know. He said it was because he was thinking something bad. I asked him why he was thinking bad thoughts. He said maybe what he was thinking wasn't all that bad. 'It's just that this shirt is the only way I can get people to talk to me,' he said."

There are rules about whom you can talk to when someone in your family has cancer. It needs to be someone who can really understand your pain and fear. Too many of us don't have even one such someone.

Recent research shows that most people have only two good friends, including family members. That is down from three in 1985. One out of four people said they had no one at all with whom they could talk about personal problems. The percentage of family members as close friends was down, too.

The researchers were startled to find such a large change in only twenty years. I'm not surprised at all by those results. Those are the same twenty years as the CIVG (computers, Internet, and video games) revolution. The electronic revolution that brings the whole world into our brains also keeps the whole world out of our hearts. We have to resort to vulgar T-shirts to get someone to talk to us.

One of the worst features of the cancer scene is isolation. One of its best features is support. But more and more, we have less and less *automatic* support, the kind that comes from family and close friends.

Being sick and alone has to be one of the worst curses this life can bring. Our chances of getting well are so much better if we are not isolated.

When I was a patient, it was not unusual for a doctor or nurse to say to me, "It would be nice if you could get friendly with that man who's in the corner chemo chair," or "the man in the back room," or "the woman with her face to the wall." They were isolated people, among the 25 percent with no one at all to talk to. They had to make do with a friend a doctor or nurse manufactured for them. But the nurses and doctors knew that a manufactured friend is better than no friend at all.

I write of this here, in the *Spouse* chapter, because this isolation trend puts great stress on families.

My wife is my best friend. When I was worried about her, concerned that she might die, I could not talk to *her* about that. We talked, of course. But my job was to share her fear, not to ask her to share mine. She felt the same way when I was the one with cancer.

Fortunately, I had other friends to whom I could talk, and so did she. But if your *only* friends are in the family, where do you get support when *they* are the ones you need to talk *about* instead of *to*?

Wives and husbands with cancer need support, especially from their spouses. Those spouses need support, too. We can't do much good for the husband or wife we love if we have no friends to share our worry with us.

One of Barbara Sher's books is titled *It's Only Too Late If You Don't Start Now*. I like that. I think it applies to making friends. If you have no one to talk to, go find someone. Call up an old classmate or teacher from high school. Go see a pastor or counselor. Pray. Ask someone at the cancer center to manufacture a friend for you. Getting your own support is a way of loving your spouse.

Now that I am the spouse of a cancer patient, I know the rule of friendship.

19. WHEN THE WORST THING POSSIBLE HAPPENS

(A CHILD OR GRANDCHILD IS THE PATIENT)

Now that I am the father and grandfather of cancer patients . . .

. . . *I trust my child.*

OUR CHILDREN WERE BORN in the early 1960s, an era when mothers were treated as invalids and fathers as interlopers. There was a special waiting room for expectant fathers, down the hall out of sight, where first-timers paced and worried while old-timers sighed heavily and told the new guys to sit down and shut up. In fact, just about everyone in the hospital told fathers to shut up and stay out of the way. We were at best a nuisance, at worst a source of germs and unwanted questions.

So I did not get to hold our first child, Mary Beth, until she was two weeks old.

There was a complication with her birth. Nothing serious, but it took two weeks to get it resolved. I was basically shut out that whole time. At the end of the two weeks a nurse wheeled Helen out of the front doors of the hospital, shoveled her onto the bench seat of our Plymouth, and placed Mary Beth on her lap.

We were parked in front of the hospital doors, but I did not care what else was going on. I grabbed that baby and held her close and admired everything about her until the door guy threatened me with mayhem if I did not get that Plymouth out of there.

That was when I realized I would never again take a nonanxious breath, that I would worry about this child every moment of my days, that this little life was more important to me than my own.

That wonder of worry has been repeated with a second daughter, with a granddaughter, with a grandson, each one as important as the others. Mary Beth was the first, however, the first to take my breath away, the first to terrify me, and that will not change.

Forty-two years after I first grabbed her and held her and knew I would always worry about her, she was diagnosed with breast cancer. It was an early diagnosis, which was good. The tumor was the fast-growing, aggressive type, which was not good. We went to Chicago to be with her for her surgery. The surgery was followed by chemotherapy and radiation, and a year of herceptin. As I write this, that year is just finished and she is doing well.

Mary Beth has made it easy on those who love her and care about her. She has given us the gift of an upbeat attitude throughout the ordeal. Her gift has made her cancer easier on her parents, but it hasn't taken away our fear. Nothing can.

There is fear when we get cancer in our own body, but there is a tragic sense of displacement, of the world in chaos, completely out of order, when your child must face cancer.

I was scared when cancer invaded my body, but I was more frightened when it invaded my daughter. That was partly because I knew what cancer does to you, what surgery and chemo do to you. Mostly it was just because she is my child. You want so much to protect your children, however young or old they may be, and sometimes you can't. You just stand there, with your hands empty and your heart heavy, and you cry.

And you trust. I am still my daughter's father, but I cannot live her life for her. My role now is to trust her. Not trust that I did a good job raising her so she'll be equal to the task she faces. That's irrelevant. Just trust her.

Now that my child has cancer, I'm learning to trust.

*. . . I go to the right place for help,
even if it's the wrong place.*

WHEN YOUR DAUGHTER HAS breast cancer, you appreciate any chance to be helpful. Running errands is a task I do pretty well, so Mary Beth sent me to the drugstore to have a prescription filled. I was not very familiar with her south side Chicago neighborhood, but how hard can it be to get around in a place that is flat and where you always know that if you go too far east, you'll end up in Lake Michigan?

Mary Beth gave me directions to a Walgreen's drugstore. I drove out of their subdivision, turned onto 95th Street, and found the drugstore right where it was supposed to be. I parked, went in, and worked my way back through greeting cards and school supplies and snack foods to the pharmacy.

As I did so, the people I met in the aisles seemed a bit surprised to see me, almost suspicious. So did the folks who sat and waited for their prescriptions to be filled. Then I got it: I was the only white person in the store.

Mary Beth lives in a mixed-race neighborhood, so I was surprised that *everyone* else was black. In most businesses on 95th Street, one sees faces of *every* color.

I went to the pharmacy window and gave the prescription to a young woman whose smock indicated she was a technician instead of a pharmacist. She was a bit suspicious, too, but that was because I wanted a prescription filled that had someone else's name on it. I explained that my daughter had breast cancer and I was doing this for her. She took care of processing the paperwork and passed it on to the pharmacist in an efficient and professional manner. But she acted like she was a bit distracted, too. Then she looked up at me and asked, with a bit of a choke in her throat, "Will she be okay?"

That, of course, was the only question I had. *Will she be okay?* It was the first time someone outside the family had shared the question and the concern with me. Will my first-born be okay? I told her I thought so. She told me she hoped so.

When I got back to Mary Beth's, I learned that I had turned the wrong way on 95th Street. I had turned east and gone into the all-black neighborhood, to the all-black Walgreen's, rather than turning west and going to the mixed-race Walgreen's, the same distance away, but in the other direction. No wonder the folks in the store looked surprised to see me; I was in the wrong place.

Except I was not, of course. I was in a place where I could get the prescription my daughter needed. I was in a place with people just like me, except for the color of our skin. I was in a place where that young woman at the pharmacy window did not see just a white man; she saw a father. She knew my daughter had to be white, but she also knew she was a young woman, just like her.

The question is the same for every parent, regardless of the color of our skin: "Will she be okay?" The question is not "Is she black? Is she white?" It is only "Will she be okay?"

I have never seen that young pharmacy technician again, but I shall always appreciate her and be thankful for her. She connected with me through that one question, sincerely asked. She voiced my concern and shared it with me. Each day, when I pray for my daughter, I pray for that young drugstore woman as well. I want her to be okay, too.

Now that I am the parent of a cancer patient, I want everyone's child to be okay.

. . . *I give a child my belt and follow.*

HE WAS TWO FEET tall and bald, with an IV line from the port in his chest to the bag on the pole. He was dressed in tan buck shoes and brown cord pants. A plaid shirt and blue pullover covered the huge and ugly scars on his abdomen. But his ensemble was not complete, and he wasn't about to let his public see him until it was.

"Belt." He pointed at mine. I had to wrap it around him twice.

Then we were off, down the hall of the children's ward, out into the main hall of the hospital, this short, bald, young babe magnet swaggering like John Wayne, with an old, bald, tall man pushing a wheeled IV pole with one hand and holding up his pants with the other while running along behind.

Joseph's liver cancer was diagnosed when he was fifteen months old. For a year he threw up everything he ate. He weighed two pounds less on his second birthday than he did on his first.

Over the fourteen months of his treatment he survived five months of the best chemotherapy protocol they could think of to shrink his tumor so it could be removed surgically. He survived three "minor" surgeries. He survived one extremely major (25 percent mortality rate) surgery to remove the tumor from his liver. That surgery was the only known cure for his particular cancer. It was not successful. The cancer spread to his lungs. They started him on another chemo protocol. In the middle of that regimen, the cancer went away.

The doctors said they had never had a chemical cure for this type of cancer. They still don't. Just because he was still on chemo when he was cured does not mean it was a chemical cure. It was a spiritual cure. It was a Joey cure.

I have no objectivity here, of course. I am gladly and unashamedly prejudiced on behalf of this boy. He is not just my grandson. He is my hero. With that disclaimer I'll still say Joseph was cured not by medicine but by spirit, by the combination of his spirit and the Holy Spirit.

Children don't all beat the odds, but they do ignore them; they ignore the odds and percentages and predictions. I don't know why they don't all beat the odds, but I know why some do. Most children live in the moment, in the right now. If there is a reason to laugh, they laugh. If there is something to learn, they learn. If there is someone to love, they love.

They don't always stay in the right *here*. Sometimes there is too much pain in the right here. But in the right *now,* they go to where there is laughter and learning and love.

Jesus said, "Unless you change and become like children, you will never enter the kingdom of heaven." There are many scholarly interpretations of this passage, from the sense of wonder and openness in children to their social and economic vulnerability. All the interpretations are probably correct. I think this one is, too: If you want to enter the kingdom of wholeness, just give a child your belt, grab your pants, and follow into the right *now* of laughter, learning, and love.

Now that I'm the grandparent of a cancer survivor,
I have no belt, but I have a hero.

. . . *I can't take the pain away.*

ONE OF THE HARDEST things about being the father or grandfather, or mother or grandmother, of a cancer patient is being unable to take the pain away. There is no kissing of boo-boos with cancer.

As I write this, I'm recovering from rotator cuff surgery. That has included daily PT for several months. The pretty young women in the hospital dungeon have mean streaks that their long blond hair doesn't hide once they get hold of your arm. They call PT physical therapy, but we patients know it as physical torture. I'm sure that if I run into my torturers at the coffee shop or mall, they won't recognize me because I won't have a twisted grimace of pain on my face, and that's the only way they have ever seen me.

One day as one of the physical terrorists was making my arm go places it definitely did not want to go, I wondered why God had not come up with a better method of letting us know when something is wrong with our bodies, a better method than pain, like a color change, or a personalized ring tone.

Actually, there are color changes in the body once in a while. If you turn blue or yellow, you know something is wrong. And there are sounds, too, like ringing in the ears or rumbling in the bowels.

But mostly the body just sticks with pain as its warning mechanism, and there's a reason for that: You have to pay attention to it. You can ignore the color yellow or a hiss or a buzz until it's too late. Pain has the advantage of making you stop right now. If your car makes a funny noise or an idiot light comes on, you'll keep driving. You wouldn't if the car gave you a whack in the nose each time instead.

The thought of a better method got my mind off and running, however.

Why not a better way of *sharing* pain? Most of us would gladly take on some of the pain of a loved one. Indeed, we want to, but we can't.

As a teacher, my wife was able to share her sick days with colleagues. If a school board could come up with a plan like that, surely God could do so as well.

On TV, I see disabled veterans of the Iraq war whose bodies are worse off than my shoulder, who must do much harder rehab. I would be willing to share their pain, but I can't. This one body is the only one I have. It's the only one on which I can do PT.

We want to help share the cancer pain of a loved one, even to death, but we can't. Each of us has only one body, and pain is not transferable.

I recall when my uncle Glen was killed in a motorcycle accident at the age of sixty-one. He was Grandma Mac's first-born. "It makes no difference how old your child is, or how old you are," she said. "When your child dies before you do, it's wrong." She was right, but it did not change the finality of Uncle Glen's death.

I have no answers here, no words of wisdom, no ideas on how to cope when a child has cancer. I know only that I stand arm in arm with every other terrified parent and grandparent.

We can share through prayer and presence and encouragement, but not in the body itself. We cannot live without one another, but there are also points beyond which we cannot go.

There is a strange paradox about life: We must have one another to create life and to give meaning to it, and yet we are always alone in life.

When a child has cancer, there's no way to kiss the boo-boo to take away the pain. Of course, kissing the boo-boo was never really intended to take away the pain, anyway. It takes away the loneliness.

Now that I'm the parent of a patient, I can't trade places to take away the pain, but I can kiss the boo-boo and take away the loneliness.

. . . We are on the same team.

TEACHING HAS THE HIGHEST turnover of any profession. The dropouts are not just young teachers who didn't know what they were getting into. I know a number of second-career ex-teachers. They wanted to make a difference, so they gave up a good living, went back to school, got certified to teach. They didn't last, in some cases not even a year.

The reasons for the high turnover are many: It's a long-hours, high-stress job that is believed by the public to have short hours and low stress. What it does have is inadequate pay, unsupportive and ineffective administrators who pay more attention to bureaucratic requirements than to what is most helpful for students, government mandates without government financing, evaluation through generic testing, bottom-line school boards, the unwillingness of taxpayers to vote for better funding, cantankerous parents, unruly students, and large classes. If that list doesn't scare you away, I don't know what will.

Yet there are people who are not scared away from teaching; some go back year after year with unflagging zeal and creativity. Like my brother Jim's wife, Millie. What is the difference? Why do so many drop out, more than any other profession, while others keep at it?

Paul J. Baker spent his career as a sociologist studying education. He was so good at it that Illinois State University designated him a distinguished professor. After a lifetime of studying teachers, Paul says there is one thing that separates the dropouts from the mainstays: the support of their peers.

He says, "Teaching is a lonely job. You are in that classroom all day all by yourself. It's a plus if you have a good principal, small classes, all the things you would expect. But the bottom line is, you can't make it if you're just alone. You need to be part of a community of other teachers who are working together."

My wife was a teacher. Each morning she and her colleagues would gather in the office to pick up their mail, drink coffee, exchange stories, and basically avoid going to their classrooms. Finally, social studies teacher Pierce Pickins would drawl, "Let's go stamp out ignorance." They would pick up their mail and their coffee and their courage and go out the door into the halls of chaos *together,* with a common goal, even though they would work alone.

When our grandson Joseph was spending his year in a hospital, 175 miles away, his four-year-old sister, Brigid, lived with Helen and me most of the time. The stresses were huge. We were old people caring for a bright, active, and upset child. In addition, we were frightened beyond words for Joey. When something happens to a grandchild, you have a double concern, for you see and feel the anguish of your children as well as the grandchildren. There were days we barely survived.

A friend gave us the best advice one can have for any hard time. She said, "Hold hands and keep putting one foot in front of the other."

If you don't have someone with whom to hold hands, do something about it. Find a support group for patients, or parents, or grandparents. If there is none, create one. It may be a group of two. That is okay. It may be only by telephone or e-mail. That is okay, but find a hand to hold and keep putting one foot in front of the other.

Now that we are grandparents, we hold hands and keep putting one foot in front of the other.

. . . *I am haunted by the night shift.*

DURING THE WEEKS THAT Joseph had to be at Children's Hospital and his father had to work and could not go along, I went to Iowa City with Joey and his mother. Helen kept his four-year-old sister, Brigid, at our house.

Kathleen never left Joey, wherever he was, including nights in the hospital. I usually spent Iowa City nights at the Ronald McDonald House a mile down the street, but sometimes it was necessary for me to spend the night in Joey's room, too.

At about two in the morning on one such night, Joey threw up. This was such a regular occurrence that we always kept extra bed gowns in the room, but he had gone through all of them. When I went to the laundry cart in the hallway to get a clean gown for him, I passed the nurse's station.

There sat the night ward clerk, holding a baby with one arm, using a foot to rock a slightly older baby in a jumpy chair, crooning a lullaby, and typing with her one free hand.

"What in the world are you doing?" I whispered.

She shrugged. "Fewer nurses on the night shift. When it gets busy, there aren't enough to keep up. So I help."

Then I remembered the head nurse, when we got our room assignment this time, saying to Katie, "We're going to put you in the far back room, because you never leave Joey." I didn't understand at the time, but now I did. They knew if they could not hear Joseph cry way back there, it was okay. Someone was with him and could call for help. That was not true with all the children.

"Where are their parents?" I asked the clerk.

"The children of single parents get sick, too," she said. "They have to work, hopefully to keep the insurance in force. If they don't have insurance, and a lot of them don't, they have to work two or three jobs."

"But where are the grandparents?"

"Sick. Old. Disabled. Dead. Florida. Keeping the other children."

I understood that. Helen and I fit all the categories but Florida. Technically we were not sick, dead, or disabled, but sometimes we felt that way.

"But these are only tiny babies and little toddlers. You can't just go off and leave them to strangers, without even enough strangers to go around."

"If you've got a better way, let us know," she said, not unkindly.

"Well, let me take this bed gown back to our room and I'll come back and hold the baby," I said. "That's the least I can do."

"Can't. You aren't staff. If you dropped it, hell to pay with lawsuits."

"I won't drop it."

"You know that. I know that. The lawyers don't know that."

"Well, let me type the stuff for you."

"Can't. Privacy issues."

"I won't tell. I won't even look. I'm old. I forget everything immediately anyway."

"You know that. I know that. The lawyers don't know that."

"Well, they should hire more staff."

"Can't. Not enough money. Already have to charge too much to those who can pay to make up for those who can't."

"Well, is there anything I can do?"

"Sure. Convince the politicians that kids need insurance, that kids with cancer are more important than their pork barrel stuff."

Now that I'm a cancer grandfather, I write letters, make telephone calls, send e-mails, march in demonstrations, and ask for adequate insurance for all children, and I ask others to join me in that task.

. . . We watch our grandson take chances.

JOSEPH WAS GIVEN SO much chemotherapy in the second year of his life that he weighed two pounds less on his second birthday than on his first. Essentially, he threw up for a year. You can't get much nourishment to grow and gain on a diet of chemo.

They told us at the hospital that the chemotherapy was so much and so strong that he would probably lose his hearing and be unable to jump. There were a lot of other warnings like that, but those are the ones I remember. I suppose I remember those because we made plans to take sign language courses and because I could not imagine anything worse for a little boy than not being able to jump. He does have some hearing loss in the upper registers, but not enough that it bothers him. He sings like a bird. And jump?

Get out of the way!

When he was a year or two beyond chemo, he was jumping off the house one day. Actually, it was a picnic table, but it looked as high as a house to worried grandparents. Also, at the same age, his mother had climbed the TV antenna and got on the roof. We got her down *before* she jumped, but we knew it was in his genes.

His grandma wanted to run and grab him before he jumped.

"We didn't get him through cancer so he could get his neck broken jumping off stuff," she said.

"Yes, we did," his mother said.

Now part of that is because she still resents it that we did not let her jump off the roof when she was four, but it's mostly because she is a wise woman and a brave mother. It takes a lot of courage to let a child be a child, especially when he has come so close to having no childhood at all.

We cannot raise our children in a padded world, as much as we would like to. We do our best to get them through the hard times, not so that they can hide from life but so they can face life, with all its challenges that have to be jumped.

Did we pray and read and worry Joey through cancer so he could take chances? Yes, we did.

Now that I'm the grandparent of a survivor, I watch him take chances. I cringe, but I watch.

. . . *T'scape*

"'SCAPE, BAMPAW. 'SCAPE!"

It was usually when his mother had slipped into the bathroom for a shower that Joey reached his arms up to me and gave me the order. I would pick him up, hold him close with my right arm, and grab his six-wheeled IV pole with my left hand, and we would escape from the third floor pediatric oncology unit.

When we were past the final doors, he would muster as much smile as he could and whisper, "Red One." We would roll down the hall to the elevator and ride down to the second floor, where the "Red One" sat in splendor in a glass case.

It was a huge red Christmas ornament with view holes in its sides. Inside was a marvelous animated winter scene: skiers gliding down a slope, skaters circling around and around on a silver pond, the twinkling lights of a village ready for Christmas. Best of all, a train circles the whole scene. Joey's tiny wasted body stiffened each time the train disappeared into the tunnel in the side of the mountain, relaxed each time its hopeful light appeared at the other end.

Each time we 'scaped, we went to the Red One, like pilgrims to Lourdes or Mecca, and we watched the skiers and skaters and the little train, the brave little train that had to risk the darkness of the tunnel time after time, until our eyes and arms grew weary. Then we would 'scape even farther.

Sometimes we would just cruise the halls, picking up chicks. I mean, that boy was the ultimate chick magnet. Young ones, old ones, it made no difference, no woman could pass him by. I did not understand it, why he got all the attention and I got none. We were both bald, after all.

He loved babies more than babes, though, so we would go to

the nursery and look at the babies. He took the babes for granted. They were just roadblocks in the hallway. But the babies were a mystery. He would stare at them, trying to figure them out, until my arms were breaking.

On our travels up and down the halls he would point out items of interest, usually "guys" and "wowas" (flowers).

Then we would 'scape to the library on the ninth floor. He was too weak and tired and haggard to play with the games and stuffed animals, but he would sit on my lap, and we would read the few books he did not have in his personal library in his room.

It was usually there that the infinitely patient nurse, Nicole Alcorn, would find us to give him a swig of medicine or attach a new bag to his IV pole. We were not supposed to 'scape his unit without signing out, telling where we would be, but I did not know that. We would just 'scape, and the ever-gracious Nicole would track us down and not say a word about our mysterious AWOL status.

Perhaps she had read the story about Jesus in his hometown and understood that sometimes a person just needs to escape for a while. Here's that story, in my translation:

The people in his hometown got so mad at him when he preached there and told the truth that they grabbed him right out of the pulpit and took him to the top of the hill on which their town was built so they could throw him off the cliff. But he passed through the midst of them and went on his way (Luke 4:16–30).

It wasn't that Jesus was afraid. He knew his life would be forfeit someday soon. That bluff in Nazareth that day just wasn't the right time or place. So he mysteriously escaped, "passing through the midst of them."

Joey escaped, too, and not just to go see the Red One with its brave little train. He had more living and loving to do, just as Jesus had more living and loving, teaching and healing to do before the place was right at Golgotha, and the time was right on that Friday we now call Good. "Then Jesus cried again with a loud voice and escaped" (Matthew 27:50, my translation).

Soon or late the time for escaping will be over for each of us, even Joey. Or will it? Perhaps death itself is the ultimate escape.

When that time comes for me, I hope Joseph is there so that he can whisper in my ear, "'Scape, Bampaw, 'scape."

. . . *I take my stance on the side of healing.*

I AM NOT SURE if it is the end of the story or its beginning, but it is where I must start.

Joseph and I were alone together in the room—a bald, exhausted tiny boy and a bald, exhausted old man. Joey was still two months short of two years.

We stood at the seventh floor window while winter darkness hovered around the hospital, hoping the helicopter would drop down upon the roof, bringing a little light to the gathering gloom, a little joy to a cheerless day. The 'copter did not come, so my little grandboy pressed close against my chest and fell asleep.

The surgery was the only cure for his type of liver cancer, they had told us, and the surgery had failed. Now they told us he would need eight more months of chemotherapy followed by surgery on both lungs followed by a liver transplant. Even then the prognosis was not good.

I did not think his twenty-two-pound body could take any more. He had already been through five months of chemo and three surgeries. He was constantly nauseated and unable to eat. He weighed less than when they had started treatments when he was fifteen months old.

I pressed that tiny body into mine until our heart beats merged. Then I spoke to the cancer:

"You know who I am. I am the grandfather. You know my rights, and you know my powers. If you must be somewhere, then come into my body, but do it quickly because you may no longer live in my grandboy."

Then his mother, my daughter, returned to the room. She took up her constant routine of weeping (while her son was sleeping) and holding and nursing and reading *The Little Engine That Could* and weeping.

Eight days later, I strapped Joey into his place in the backseat of my car for the long ride home. As I leaned over to place this skinny, sunken-eyed, sick, scrawny-necked bald little boy into his car seat, so ill from the chemo that he had not eaten for a week and probably would not for another, that was when I knew. It seemed ludicrous. He looked so tired, so worn, like a little war orphan who had been bombed far too long, but that was when I knew: The cancer was gone. I dared not tell anyone, but I knew.

WHEN WE RETURNED IN three weeks, the tests confirmed it. The cancer was gone.

The question immediately arises: Why Joey? Other people have loved other children as much, prayed for them as hard, hoped for them as eagerly and anxiously. If Joseph experienced a spiritual cure, because of the prayers of so many people, why are not other children cured?

I have no answer at all for that. I myself have prayed hard and long for children who were not cured. Prayer is the only healing power of which we ask perfection. Surgery does not always work, but we do not stop using it. The same with chemotherapy and penicillin and every wonder drug. They are all imperfect, but we keep using them because we know that they work sometimes. My wife is currently taking a medicine that is very helpful to her. Her doctor says, "We don't know how or why this medicine works for this condition. We simply know that it does."

So it is with prayer. So it is with hope. My prayers are not always answered, but I dare not stop praying, because *sometimes* they are answered. I do not know how or why prayer works, but I know it does. However imperfect our means of healing, I know that if I have an opportunity to take my stance on the side of healing, that is where I want to be. If prayer is the only hammer I have, that is the one I'll swing.

Now that I am the parent and grandparent of cancer patients, I take my stance on the side of healing.

BIBLIOGRAPHY

HERE IS A LIST of books mentioned in the meditations.

Anderson, Greg. *The Cancer Conqueror.* Kansas City: Andrews McMeel, 1988.

Borysenko, Joan. *Minding the Body, Mending the Mind.* New York: Bantam, 1988.

Borysenko, Joan. *Guilt Is the Teacher, Love Is the Lesson.* New York: Warner Books, 1990.

Bradbury, Ray. *The Martian Chronicles.* New York: Doubleday, 1950.

Cousins, Norman. *Head First: The Biology of Hope.* New York: E.P. Dutton, 1989.

Dooley, Tom. *The Night They Burned the Mountain.* New York: Farrar, Straus, & Cudahy, 1960.

Hill, Albert F., with Paul K. Hamilton and Lynn Ringer. *I'm a Patient, Too.* New York: Nick Lyons Books, 1986.

Hillerman, Tony. *Talking God.* New York: Harper & Row, 1989.

Klein, Allen. *The Whole Mirth Catalog.* San Francisco: Allen Klein.

McFarland, John Robert. *The Strange Calling: Stories of Ministry.* Macon, GA: Smyth & Helwys, 1999.

Palencia, Elaine Fowler. *Brier Country: Stories from Blue Valley.* Columbia: University of Missouri Press, 2000.

Palencia, Elaine Fowler. *The Dailyness of It.* Louisville, KY: Grex Press, 2002.

Ryan, Regina Sara. *The Fine Art of Recuperation: A Guide to Surviving and Thriving After Illness, Accident, or Surgery.* Los Angeles: Jeremy P. Tarcher, 1989.

Sher, Barbara. *It's Only Too Late If You Don't Start Now.* New York: Delacorte Press, 1988.

Shideler, Mary McDermott. *In Search of the Spirit.* New York: Ballantine, 1985.

Siegel, Bernie S. *Love, Medicine, & Miracles.* New York: Harper & Row, 1986.

Siegel, Bernie S. *Peace, Love, & Healing.* New York: Harper & Row, 1989.